THE Ultimate FODMAP Cookbook

150 deliciously **easy recipes** to **soothe** your gut and **nourish** your body

Vermilion
LONDON

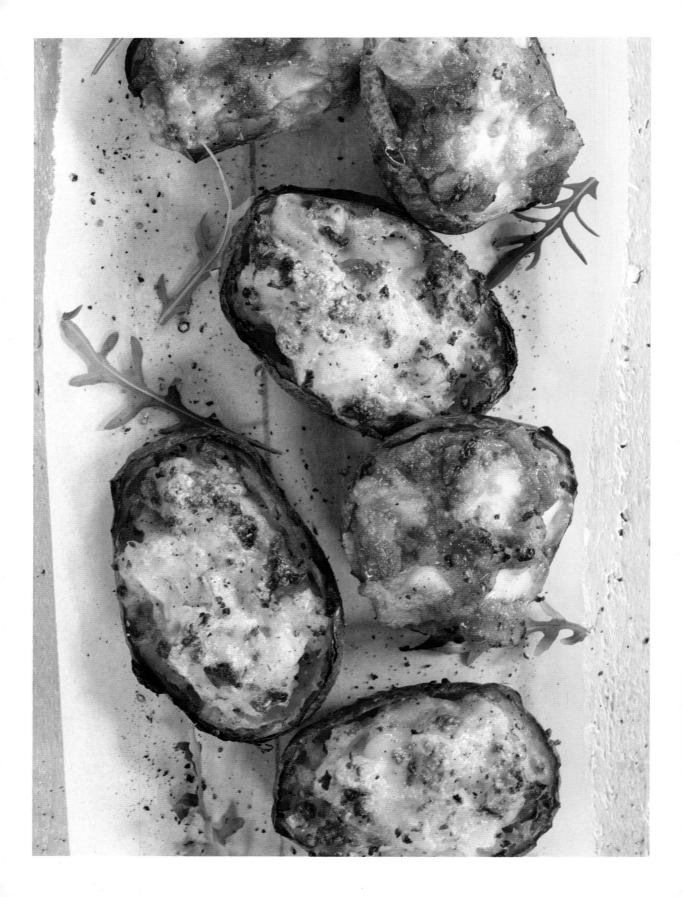

XC

THE
Ultir
FOD
Cool

150 deliciously
your gut and

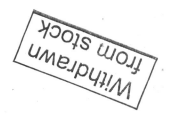

10 9 8 7 6 5 4 3 2 1

Vermilion, an imprint of Ebury Publishing,
20 Vauxhall Bridge Road,
London, SW1V 2SA

Vermilion is part of the Penguin Random House group of companies whose
addresses can be found at global.penguinrandomhouse.com

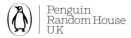
Penguin
Random House
UK

Text: Heather Thomas
Photography: Howard Shooter
Design: Maru Studio
Food Styling: Moo Jevons
Recipe Editor: Becci Woods

First published by Vermilion in 2017

www.penguin.co.uk

A CIP catalogue record for this book is available from the British Library

ISBN: 9781785041419

Printed and bound in China by Toppan Leefung

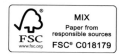

MIX
Paper from
responsible sources
FSC® C018179

Penguin Random House is committed to a sustainable
future for our business, our readers and our planet. This
book is made from Forest Stewardship Council® certified
paper.

The information in this book has been compiled by way of general guidance in
relation to the specific subjects addressed, but is not a substitute and not to be relied
on for medical, healthcare, pharmaceutical or other professional advice on specific
circumstances and in specific locations. So far as the author is aware the information
given is correct and up to date as at December 2017. Practice, laws and regulations
all change, and the reader should obtain up-to-date professional advice on any such
issues. The author and publishers disclaim, as far as the law allows, any liability arising
directly or indirectly from the use, or misuse, of the information contained in this book.

CONTENTS

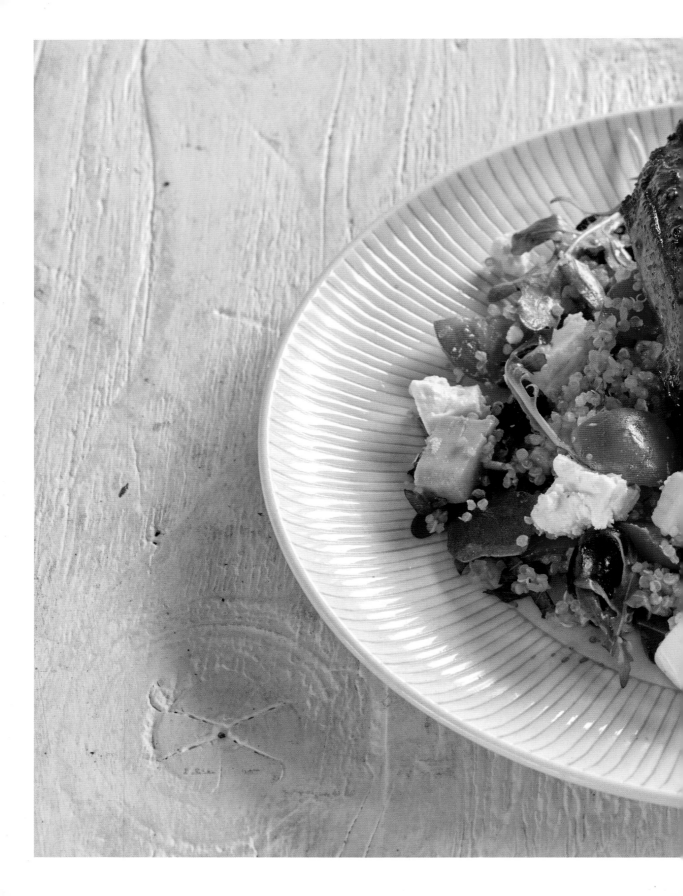

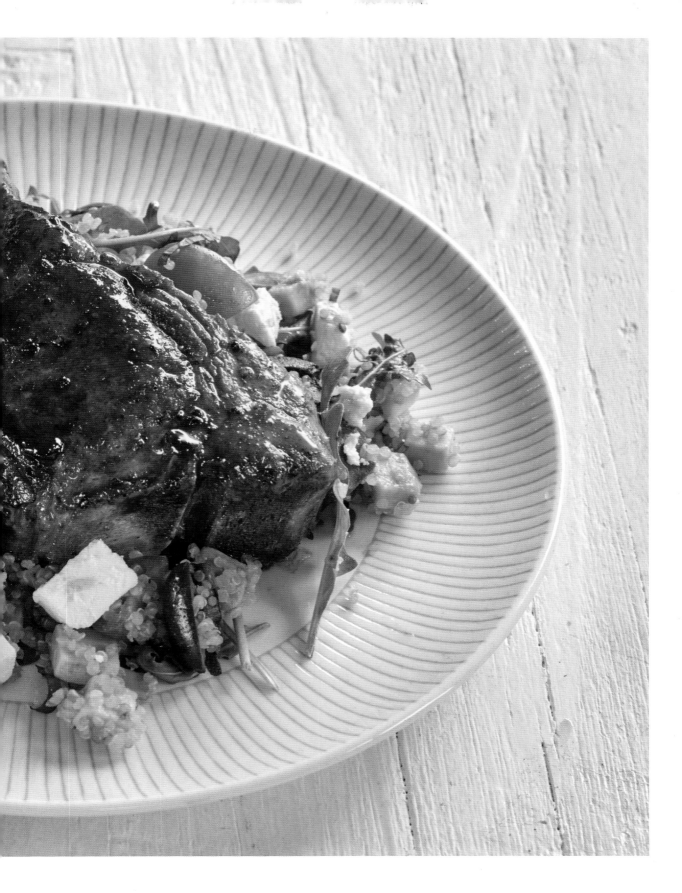

INTRODUCTION

The low FODMAP diet is a scientifically proven and effective way of managing and reducing the symptoms of IBS (irritable bowel syndrome) and other bowel diseases and disorders, including coeliac disease, ulcerative colitis and Crohn's disease. If you suffer from these digestive problems, eating the low FODMAP way won't cure you but it will ease your symptoms and help make you feel healthier and better – and you can still enjoy your food. It's simple once you identify your trigger foods and cut them out of your everyday diet.

FODMAP is an acronym that stands for a group of poorly absorbed short-chain carbohydrates: Fermentable Oligosaccharides, Disaccharides, Monosaccharides And Polypols. When these are fermented in the colon, they can cause discomfort, bloating, wind and diarrhoea. Cutting them out of your diet altogether, or reducing the amount you consume, can bring relief or even eliminate the symptoms altogether. To get the best results, you should follow the diet with a specialist dietitian; talk to your doctor about a referral.

On the FODMAP diet, some foods are safe to eat while others should only be eaten in moderation or avoided completely. Look at the charts on pages 12–15 to find out which foods you can eat freely and which you should restrict (maximum amounts are stated). It looks a bit complicated at first, but you'll soon get the hang of it as you start cooking and putting it into practice.

The recipes featured in this book are all easy to make and don't require any specialist skills or techniques. They will help you to navigate the diet and teach you how to cook without everyday ingredients, including onions, garlic, flour and pasta that contain gluten or dairy foods with lactose. There's lots of choice and whatever your food preferences you'll find delicious, healthy recipes that you can't wait to try out.

COOKING & EATING
THE FODMAP WAY

Here are some practical tips and advice to help you cook and eat the FODMAP way. It's not complicated or time-consuming and the guidelines will soon become second nature to you.

- Use garlic-infused oil to add flavour to a sauce, salad dressing, stir-fry or a savoury dish.

- Add some snipped chives when you're cooking or sprinkle them over the finished dish just before serving for a mild oniony flavour.

- To intensify the onion flavour, you can use the chopped or sliced green parts of leeks and spring onions (scallions) in small quantities.

- To intensify the garlic flavour in salads, you can rub a cut clove around the inside of the bowl before adding the salad leaves and vegetables.

- Always use onion-free stock cubes and bouillon powder – check the labels carefully before purchasing.

- Check the labels for hidden onion or garlic on spice blends, gravy, marinades, sauces, potato crisps (chips) and rice crackers.

- Use FODMAP-friendly seasonings and flavourings instead of onion and garlic: herbs, spices, lemongrass, sumac, poppy and sesame seeds, vanilla, etc.

- You can make great low FODMAP curries using strongly flavoured ingredients such as galangal, Thai fish sauce, kaffir lime leaves, curry leaves, ground spices, fresh root ginger and coconut milk. You won't miss the onion and garlic.

- If you are lactose-intolerant, choose lactose-free alternatives to milk, yoghurt, cheese and other dairy products.

- Eat gluten-free bread and pasta and use gluten-free flour when cooking.

- Check the labels on food products for wheat and gluten. You may be surprised at the number of food items that contain them, e.g. canned soup, bottled sauces, dressings and marinades and processed meat.

- Soy products can be a little confusing on a FODMAP diet – some can contain high levels of oligosaccharides, but manufacturing processes will greatly reduce the FODMAP content. As a rule of thumb, tempeh, firm tofu (as opposed to silken), miso and soy lecithin are low-FODMAP. Soy milk made from soy protein is OK too, but watch out for soy milk made from whole or hulled soybeans.

FODMAP CHARTS

LOW FODMAP: EAT FREELY

MEAT & POULTRY
Bacon
Beef
Chicken
Ham
Lamb
Pork
Prosciutto
Turkey

FISH & SHELLFISH
All fresh fish
All fresh shellfish
Canned tuna

VEGETARIAN PROTEIN
Quorn food products, e.g. mince
Tempeh
Tofu

VEGETABLES
Alfalfa
Aubergines (eggplants)
Bamboo shoots
Bean sprouts
Carrots
Celeriac (celery root)
Chicory
Chilli
Chinese leaves (Chinese cabbage)
Chives – use instead of onion
Courgettes (zucchini)
Cucumber
Endive
Ginger
Green beans
Kale
Leeks – green leaves only
Lettuce
Marrow

Olives
Pak choi (bok choy)
Parsley
Parsnips
Peppers (bell peppers)
Potatoes
Pumpkin
Radicchio
Radishes
Rocket (arugula)
Seaweed/nori
Spinach
Spring onions (scallions) – green
    leaves only
Squash – all varieties except
    butternut
Swede (rutabaga)
Swiss chard
Tomatoes, fresh and canned
    (not cherry)
Turnips
Water chestnuts
Watercress
Yams

FRUIT
Ackee
Bananas
Blueberries
Breadfruit
Clementines
Cranberries
Grapefruit
Guava
Kiwi fruit
Lemons
Limes
Mangoes
Melons – all except watermelon
Oranges

Papayas (pawpaw)
Passion fruit
Raspberries
Rhubarb
Strawberries
Tamarind

DRIED FRUIT
Banana chips
Cranberries
Currants
Papaya (pawpaw)
Pineapple
Raisins
Sultanas (golden raisins)

GRAINS & CEREALS
Arrowroot
Breadcrumbs – gluten-free only
Buckwheat – flour and noodles
  & soba noodles
Corn chips/tortillas/flakes
Cornflour (cornstarch)
Cornmeal
Millet
Oatcakes
Oats – porridge and oat bran
Polenta
Popcorn
Porridge
Potato flour
Pretzels
Quinoa
Rice – brown, white, basmati;
  noodles & vermicelli; flour;
  rice bran
Rice cakes
Sorghum
Soy flour
Tapioca – including flour

Wheat-free or gluten-free pasta
Wheat-free or gluten-free bread,
  e.g. corn, oat, rice bread,
  potato flour bread
Xanthan gum

NUTS & SEEDS
Chia seeds
Coconut
Flax seeds/linseed
Poppy seeds
Sesame seeds

STORE CUPBOARD
Almond extract
Artificial sweeteners – not
  ending in 'ol', e.g. aspartame,
  stevia
Asafoetida powder (onion
  substitute)
Baking powder – gluten-free
  if on gluten-free diet
Bicarbonate of soda
  (baking soda)
Capers
Chocolate – dark only
Chocolate spread
Cocoa powder
Coffee
Fish sauce (nam pla)
Gelatine
Ghee
Golden syrup (corn syrup) –
  unless high-fructose
Herbs
Jam – fructose-free only
Maple syrup
Marmite
Mayonnaise (plain)
Miso paste

Molasses
Mustard
Oils – all, including garlic-infused,
  if wished, for flavouring
Oyster sauce
Salt
Shrimp paste
Soy sauce – gluten-free if
  on gluten-free diet
Spices
Stock – onion-free only
Sugar
Sweet & sour sauce
Tamari
Tamarind paste
Tea
Vanilla extract
Vinegar
Wasabi
Worcestershire sauce

DAIRY
Butter
Cheese – blue cheese,
  Brie, Camembert, Cheddar,
  cottage, feta, goat's, mozzarella
  (buffalo for lactose-intolerant),
  Parmesan, Swiss
Eggs
Margarine
Milk – whole/semi-skimmed/
  skimmed or lactose-free,
  soya milk (if tolerated)
  or suitable plant-based,
  e.g. almond milk
Sorbet – made from low-
  FODMAP fruit
Yoghurt – lactose-free or
  Greek yoghurt

EAT IN MODERATION (IF TOLERATED)

VEGETABLES

Asparagus – 3 spears max

Avocados – ¼ max

Beetroot (beets) – ½ medium

Broccoli – 150g/½ cup max

Brussels sprouts – 2 max

Butternut squash –60g/2oz
(¼ cup) max

Cabbage, Savoy – 150g/5oz
(1 cup) max

Cauliflower – in small amounts
only

Celery – in small amounts,
e.g. 1 stalk

Fennel – 100g/3½oz max

Mangetout (snow peas) – 10
pods max

Mushrooms – in small amounts
only

Peas – 60g/2oz (generous ¼ cup)
max

Sweetcorn – ½ cob max

Sweet potato – 90g/generous
3oz (scant ½ cup) max

Tomatoes, sun-dried – 4 pieces
max

LEGUMES

Canned chickpeas: 20g/scant 1oz
(⅛ cup), well rinsed, max

Canned lentils: 20g/scant 1oz
(⅛ cup), well rinsed, max

FRUIT

Grapes – 10 max

Pineapple – in small amounts,
e.g. 1 slice

Pomegranates – seeds from ½
small

GRAINS & CEREALS

Oatmeal – 60g/2oz (½ cup) max

NUTS & SEEDS

Almonds – 10 max

Brazil nuts – 1 handful max

Chestnuts – 1 handful max

Hazelnuts – 10 max

Macadamia nuts – 1 handful max

Peanuts – 1 handful max

Pecans – 10 max

Pine nuts – 10 max

Walnuts – 1 handful max

Seeds – most kinds (hemp,
pumpkin, sunflower, etc.)
1 handful max

STORE CUPBOARD

Chocolate – 3 squares milk or
white max

Chutney – 1 tbsp max

Peanut butter – 2 tbsp max

Pesto sauce – less than 1 tbsp
max

Seed butters – 2 tbsp max

DAIRY

Cream – 120ml/4fl oz (½ cup)
max

Cream cheese – 50g/2oz (¼ cup)
max

Ricotta – 2tbsp

HIGH FODMAP: DON'T EAT!

MEAT
All processed meats, such as sausages, chorizo, salamis and pepperoni
Sausages

VEGETABLES
Artichokes
Broad beans
Garlic
Leeks (white stems)
Okra
Onions
Shallots
Soybeans
Spring onions (white stems)
Sugar snap peas
Tomatoes, cherry

VEGETARIAN PROTEIN
Some soy products (unless tolerated) (see note on page 9)

LEGUMES
Chickpeas – cooked from dry
Falafel
Lentils – cooked from dry
All other legumes, dried or canned, e.g. kidney, black, cannellini, butterbeans (lima beans), broad beans (fava), haricot (navy), aduki, soy, etc.

FRUIT
Apples
Apricots
Blackberries
Cherries
Dates
Figs
Goji berries
Lychees
Nectarines
Peaches
Pears
Persimmons
Plums
Watermelon

DRIED FRUIT
Prunes

GRAINS & CEREALS (CHECK LABELS)
All wheat products – including biscuits, bread, breakfast cereals, cakes, cereal bars, cookies, croissants, crumpets, muffins, naan, pitta, pumpernickel, scones, etc.
Bran – wheat bran only, including wheat-bran cereals
Breadcrumbs – containing wheat or rye
Bulgur wheat
Couscous
Flour – wheat and rye
Freekeh
Granola – containing wheat or rye
Muesli – containing wheat or rye flakes
Noodles – egg and udon
Pasta – made from wheat, including durum wheat
Pastry – made from wheat or rye flour
Rye bread and crackers
Semolina – including gnocchi
Spelt

NUTS
Cashews
Pistachios

STORE CUPBOARD
Agave syrup
Artificial sweeteners
Baked beans
Carob powder
Fructose – including high-fructose corn syrup
Honey
Hummus
Jam – unless fructose-free
Relishes and pickles
Stock cubes – unless onion-free
Tahini

DAIRY
Buttermilk
Cheese – halloumi (unless tolerated)
Custard
Ice cream
Kefir
Milk – cow's, goat's, sheep's unless lactose-free, for some people
Soured cream
Yoghurt – unless lactose-free or Greek, for some people

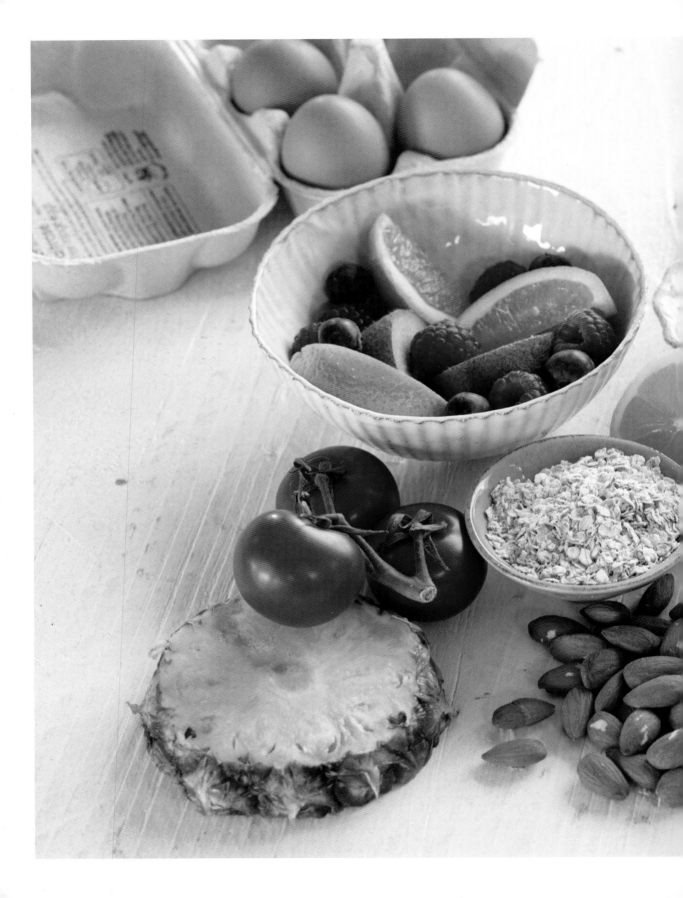

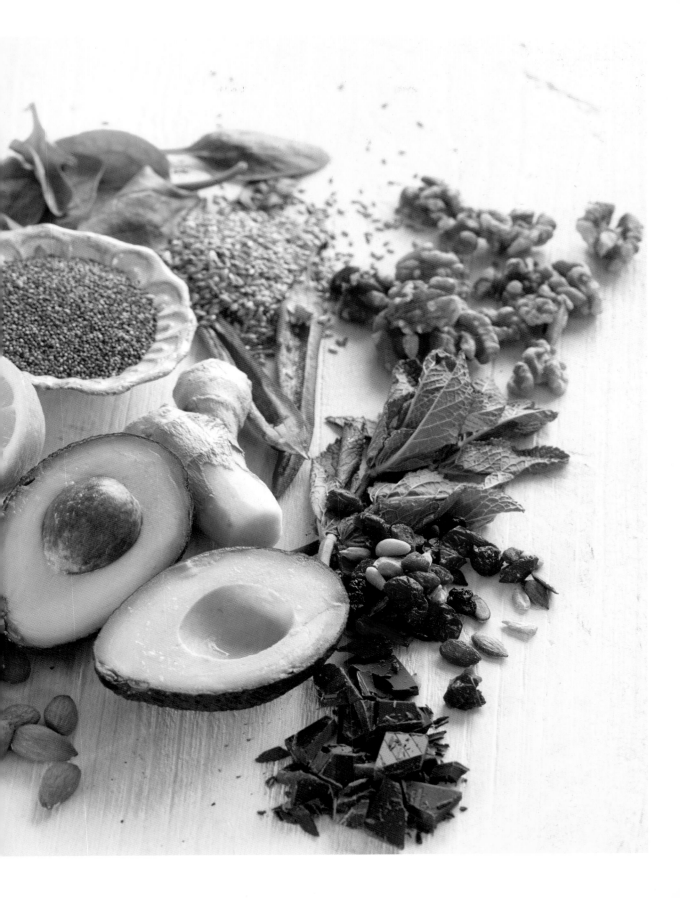

BREAKFASTS
&
BRUNCHES

CHIA SEED PORRIDGE

Chia seeds are a great source of protein, vitamins and minerals and have the ability to absorb liquids and swell up to 15 times their original size. This 'porridge' can be prepared quickly and easily the night before eating, ready to top with yoghurt, fruit, nuts and seeds just before serving.

SERVES 4
PREP: 10 MIN, PLUS OVERNIGHT CHILLING
COOK: 1–2 MIN

2 bananas, mashed

8 tbsp chia seeds

600ml/1 pint (2½ cups) unsweetened almond or coconut milk

grated zest of 1 orange

60g/2oz (¼ cup) coconut yoghurt or lactose-free yoghurt

maple syrup, for drizzling (optional)

raspberries, strawberries or blueberries, for topping

FOR THE TOASTED NUT & SEED TOPPING

2 tbsp chopped almonds, walnuts or hazelnuts

2 tbsp flax or pumpkin seeds

2 tbsp coconut flakes

1. Put the mashed bananas and chia seeds in a large bowl and whisk in the nut milk until well combined, smooth and lump free. Set aside for 3 minutes and whisk in the orange zest. Cover the bowl and chill overnight in the refrigerator.

2. The following morning, when the mixture has thickened to a tapioca-like porridge, divide it between 4 bowls and add a spoonful of coconut yoghurt to each one.

3. Heat a small frying pan (skillet) over a medium heat and dry-fry the chopped nuts and seeds, tossing them gently once or twice, for 1–2 minutes until golden. Remove from the pan immediately and stir in the coconut flakes.

4. Sprinkle the toasted nuts and seeds over the porridge. Drizzle with maple syrup (if using) and top with fresh berries.

OR YOU CAN TRY THIS...

- Vary the topping with chopped pecans or pine nuts; dried cranberries, raisins or banana chips; shelled hemp seeds or sunflower seeds.

- Flavour the porridge with vanilla or almond extract or a pinch of ground cinnamon or nutmeg.

- If you don't like thick porridge, you can thin it with some more nut milk or even a little orange juice.

HIGH-PROTEIN QUINOA PORRIDGE

This porridge is a warming and satisfying way to start the day. It keeps well, so you can put some aside, sealed in a container in the fridge and reheat it the following day in the microwave or in a small pan with some milk or water.

SERVES 4
PREP: 5 MIN
COOK: 15–20 MIN

110g/4oz (generous ½ cup) quinoa flakes

110g/4oz (generous 1 cup) rolled oats

a pinch of salt

vanilla seeds from 1 vanilla pod (bean)

600ml/1 pint (2½ cups) coconut milk or unsweetened almond milk or lactose-free milk

110g/4oz (½ cup) coconut yoghurt or lactose-free yoghurt

molasses sugar, for sprinkling (optional)

seeds of 1 small pomegranate

1. Put the quinoa flakes, rolled oats and salt in a saucepan with the vanilla seeds and milk.

2. Stir well over a low to medium until the porridge starts to thicken. Simmer gently for 10 minutes until thick and smooth. If it's too thick for your taste, thin it with a little water or more milk.

3. Stir in the yoghurt and divide between 4 bowls or serve the porridge with the yoghurt on top. Sprinkle with the molasses sugar (if using) and pomegranate seeds.

OR YOU CAN TRY THIS...

- Instead of vanilla seeds, use vanilla extract or add some ground spices (ginger, nutmeg, cinnamon, cloves or cardamom).

- For a chocolate-flavoured porridge, stir in 1 tablespoon cocoa powder and sweeten with sugar or maple syrup.

- Stir in 2 tablespoons chia seeds just before serving.

- Sprinkle the porridge with fresh berries, stewed rhubarb, sliced banana, coconut flakes or chopped almonds.

MATCHA & CHIA SEED POWERPOTS

Another breakfast that you can prepare the night before – perfect for early risers who are rushing to get off to work. And because it can be made in a screwtop jar, you can even pop one into your bag to take with you. The matcha adds a delicate flavour and amazing fresh green colour.

SERVES 4
PREP: 15 MIN, PLUS OVERNIGHT CHILLING

8 tbsp chia seeds

a few drops of vanilla extract

500ml/18fl oz (2¼ cups) unsweetened almond milk

1 tsp good-quality matcha powder

1 tbsp maple syrup

1 papaya (pawpaw) or small mango, peeled, deseeded and diced

4 tbsp thick Greek yoghurt or lactose-free yoghurt

110g/4oz (1 cup) fresh blueberries

4 tbsp chopped almonds or hazelnuts

1. Whisk the chia seeds, vanilla and almond milk in a bowl to distribute the seeds evenly throughout.

2. In another bowl, mix the matcha powder and maple syrup until well blended and smooth, then stir into the chia mixture with the diced fruit.

3. Divide between 4 glass pots, screwtop jam jars or mugs and screw on the lids or cover with cling film (plastic wrap).

4. Chill in the refrigerator overnight until all the liquid is absorbed and the mixture swells and has a jelly-like texture.

5. The following day, top each pot with a spoonful of yoghurt and sprinkle with blueberries and chopped nuts just before serving.

OR YOU CAN TRY THIS...
- Top the powerpots with raspberries, sliced strawberries or banana.

- Use reduced-fat coconut milk instead of almond milk and top with coconut yoghurt.

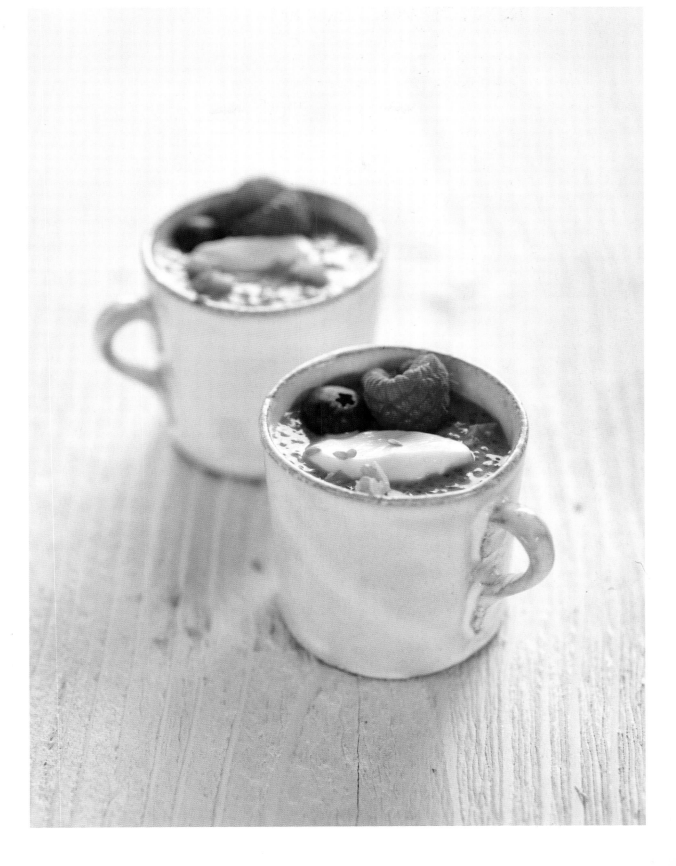

GRANOLA BREAKFAST BOWL

You can make double the quantity of granola and store it in an airtight container for up to a month. Eat it with yoghurt and fresh or stewed FODMAP-friendly fruit, or plain with soya, nut or lactose-free milk.

SERVES 4
PREP: 15 MIN
COOK: 20–25 MIN

450g/1lb young pink rhubarb stems, trimmed and cut into chunks

grated zest and juice of 1 large orange

3 tbsp soft brown sugar

seeds of 1 vanilla pod (bean)

4 tbsp 0% fat Greek yoghurt or lactose-free yoghurt

FOR THE GRANOLA:

30g/1oz (2 tbsp) coconut oil

2 tbsp maple syrup

110g/4oz (generous 1 cup) rolled oats

2 tbsp roughly chopped walnuts or hazelnuts

3 tbsp flaked almonds

30g/1oz (scant ¼ cup) sunflower seeds

30g/1oz (scant ¼ cup) pumpkin seeds

2 tbsp sesame seeds

2 tbsp dried cranberries

a pinch of ground cinnamon

> **TIP**
> Remove the vanilla seeds by splitting the pod (bean) lengthways and then scraping them out with the point of a sharp knife.

1. Preheat the oven to 170°C, 325°F, gas mark 3.

2. Make the granola: heat the coconut oil and maple syrup in a pan set over a low heat until the coconut oil melts. Stir in the oats, nuts, seeds, cranberries and cinnamon, making sure everything is well coated. Remove from the heat.

3. Pour the mixture in a thin layer over a large baking tray (cookie sheet), spreading it out evenly. Bake in the preheated oven for 15–20 minutes, stirring once or twice, until golden brown and crisp. Set aside to cool.

4. Meanwhile, arrange the rhubarb in a single layer in a roasting tin (pan). Sprinkle with the grated orange zest and juice, brown sugar and vanilla seeds. Tuck the empty vanilla pod between the rhubarb chunks.

5. Cover with kitchen foil and bake in the preheated oven for 15–20 minutes until tender but not mushy – the rhubarb should hold its shape. Allow to cool and discard the vanilla pod.

6. Divide the rhubarb between 4 glass jars or bowls and cover with the granola. Top with a spoonful of yoghurt.

OR YOU CAN TRY THIS...

- Vary the seeds in the granola: try shelled flax and hemp seeds.

- Add coconut flakes instead of almonds.

- Instead of rhubarb, serve the granola with a compôte of strawberries, blueberries or raspberries.

OVERNIGHT OAT & FRUIT POTS

Make these little pots in the evening and chill in the fridge overnight to enable the yoghurt and milk to soften the oats. They make an easy and delicious breakfast with minimal fuss and effort.

SERVES 4
PREP: 10 MIN, PLUS OVERNIGHT CHILLING

500ml/18lb oz (2 cups) 0% fat Greek yoghurt
   or lactose-free yoghurt

120ml/4fl oz (½ cup) skimmed milk, soy milk,
   nut milk or lactose-free milk,

8 tbsp porridge oats

3 tbsp mixed seeds, e.g. pumpkin, sunflower,
   linseed (flax seed), chia

2 tbsp chopped pecans, almonds or hazelnuts

400g/14oz (2 cups) mixed berries, e.g. strawberries,
   raspberries, blueberries

1. Mix most of the Greek yoghurt with the milk, porridge oats, seeds and nuts.

2. Divide the mixture between 4 shallow glass jars or clear containers and cover with half of the berries. Top with the remaining yoghurt and the rest of the berries.

3. Cover and leave in the fridge overnight. Eat for breakfast the following morning.

OR YOU CAN TRY THIS...

- If you have a sweet tooth, you can stir a spoonful of maple syrup into the yoghurt mixture or drizzle some over the berries just before eating.

- Flavour the yoghurt with a few drops of vanilla extract or some grated orange zest.

- Vary the fruit according to what's available or seasonal: use kiwi, melon, papaya (pawpaw), orange or clementine segments. Or top with sliced banana just before serving.

DETOX FRUIT & VEG SMOOTHIE

This cleansing green smoothie is highly nutritious and a great way to kickstart your day. Just put all the ingredients in a blender and blitz until smooth – nothing could be simpler.

SERVES 2
PREP: 10 MIN

2 slices fresh pineapple, chopped

2 bananas, peeled

1 kiwi fruit, peeled and sliced

2 handfuls baby spinach leaves

2.5cm/1in piece fresh root ginger, peeled and chopped

480ml/16fl oz (2 cups) almond milk or soya milk

2 tsp linseeds (flax seeds)

2 tsp chopped almonds

1. Put the pineapple, bananas, kiwi fruit, spinach and ginger in a blender or food processor. Add the almond milk and seeds.

2. Holding the lid of the blender firmly in place, blitz until everything is well combined and smooth. If the smoothie is too thick for your taste, add a little water to get the desired consistency.

3. Pour the smoothie into 2 glasses, sprinkle with the almonds and serve. Alternatively, transfer to a jug and chill in the fridge for 1 hour – no longer or the banana will discolour.

OR YOU CAN TRY THIS...

- Instead of pineapple and kiwi fruit, add some diced mango and strawberries.
- Use fresh kale instead of spinach.
- Add a scoop of protein powder (vegetable or lactose-free).
- For a fresh citrusy flavour and extra vitamin C, add the juice of 1 lime.

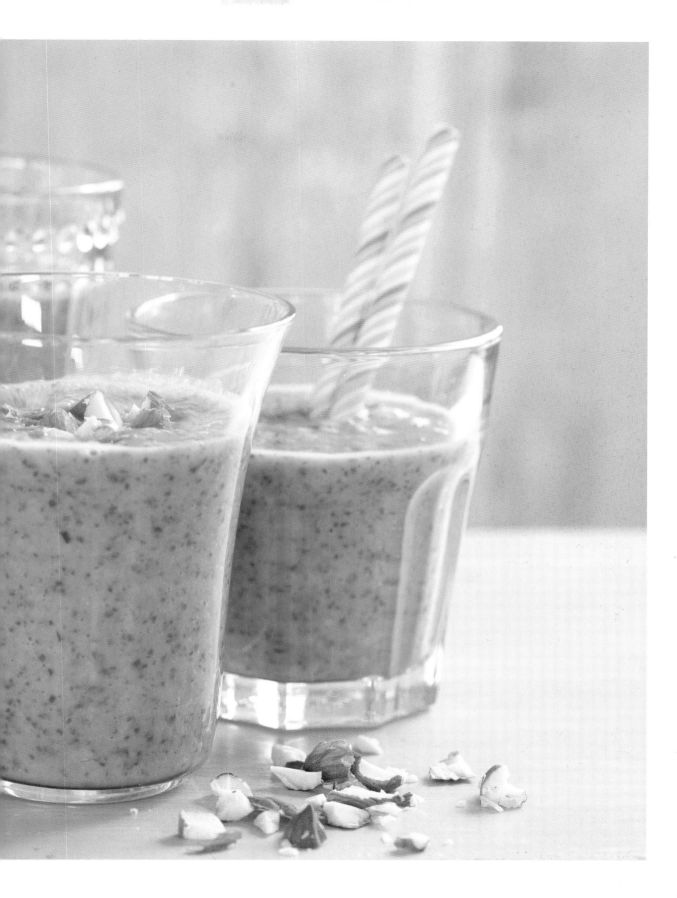

FRUITY BREAKFAST BARS

These breakfast bars are really quick and easy to make. Packed with nutrients and high in energy, they are low GI (glycaemic index), which means they are digested and absorbed slowly into your bloodstream without causing a surge in your blood sugar levels. This helps to prevent mid-morning hunger and keeps you going until lunchtime without snacking.

MAKES 12 BARS
PREP: 10 MIN
COOK: 15–20 MIN

300g/10½oz (generous 3½ cups) rolled oats

110g/4oz (¾ cup) dried cranberries

150g/5oz (1 cup) raisins

30g/1oz (scant ¼ cup) sunflower seeds

2 tbsp sesame seeds

2 tbsp chopped almonds

2 tsp ground cinnamon

1 tbsp coconut oil

1 tbsp maple syrup

a few drops of vanilla extract

2 bananas, mashed

1. Preheat the oven to 180°C, 350°F, gas mark 4.

2. Mix the oats, cranberries, raisins, seeds, almonds and cinnamon in a bowl. Melt the coconut oil in a small pan and stir in the maple syrup and vanilla. Mix into the dry ingredients with the mashed bananas.

3. Transfer the mixture to a baking tray (pan), lined with parchment paper, and level the top. Bake in the preheated oven for 15–20 minutes until golden brown.

4. Remove from the oven and cut into 12 bars while warm. Set aside and leave to cool. Store in an airtight container.

OR YOU CAN TRY THIS...

- Add a couple of spoonfuls of chopped hazelnuts to the mixture.

- Stir a tablespoon of crunchy peanut butter into the melted coconut oil.

- Try adding a few cacao nibs or some chia seeds or linseeds (flax seeds).

- If you don't have coconut oil use sunflower instead.

NO-PASTRY MINI BREAKFAST 'QUICHES'

These little individual 'quiches' can be made in advance and eaten warm for breakfast or taken to work as a packed lunch. Without a pastry case (shell), they are low in calories and gluten-free, making them a healthy snack (approximately 100 calories per quiche).

SERVES 4
PREP: 10 MIN
COOK: 25–30 MIN

1 tbsp olive oil, plus extra
    for brushing

1 red or yellow (bell) pepper,
    deseeded and chopped

2 tomatoes, diced

85g/3oz mushrooms, diced

a handful of baby spinach leaves

2 medium free-range eggs

4 tbsp skimmed milk, lactose-free
    milk, soya milk or nut milk

a small bunch of chives, snipped

100g/3½oz (scant ½ cup) low-fat
    cottage cheese

salt and freshly ground black
    pepper

1. Preheat the oven to 190°C, 375°F, gas mark 5.

2. Heat the oil in a frying pan (skillet) over a medium heat. Add the red or yellow (bell) pepper and cook for 4–5 minutes until it starts to soften. Stir in the tomatoes, mushrooms and spinach and cook for 2 minutes. Remove the pan from the heat.

3. Lightly brush 4 non-stick muffin pans with oil and divide the vegetable mixture between them.

4. Beat the eggs and milk together in a bowl. Stir in the chives and cottage cheese, and season with salt and pepper. Pour the mixture over the vegetables in the muffin pans.

5. Bake in the preheated oven for 15–20 minutes or until well risen, golden brown and firm to the touch.

6. Eat the mini quiches immediately or set aside to cool and then store in an airtight container in the fridge for breakfast.

OR YOU CAN TRY THIS...

- Use curly kale instead of spinach.

- Mix some diced lean ham or chopped prosciutto into the vegetable mixture.

- Instead of cottage cheese, use grated Cheddar or Parmesan.

- Make the quiches spicy with a pinch of dried chilli (hot pepper) flakes.

SPICY CHIA SCRAMBLED EGG WRAPS

Chia seeds can be added to scrambled eggs to make these Mexican-style wraps – perfect for a weekend breakfast or brunch.

SERVES 4
PREP: 10 MIN
COOK: 8–10 MIN

1 tbsp olive oil

1 red chilli, diced

4 juicy tomatoes, roughly chopped

6 medium free-range eggs

3 tbsp chia seeds

a small bunch of chives, snipped

4 cornmeal tortilla wraps

a handful of baby spinach leaves

1 small ripe avocado, peeled, stoned (pitted) and diced

juice of ½ lime

salt and freshly ground black pepper

1. Heat the olive oil in a non-stick frying pan (skillet), add the chilli and tomatoes and cook over a medium heat for 2–3 minutes.

2. Meanwhile, beat the eggs with the chia seeds and chives. Season lightly with salt and pepper. Pour the egg mixture into the pan and stir with a wooden spoon until the eggs start to scramble and set.

3. Heat the tortilla wraps in a low oven or on a griddle pan.

4. Toss the spinach and avocado in the lime juice and scatter over the warm tortillas. Spoon the scrambled egg mixture on top and roll up or fold over to make parcels. Serve immediately.

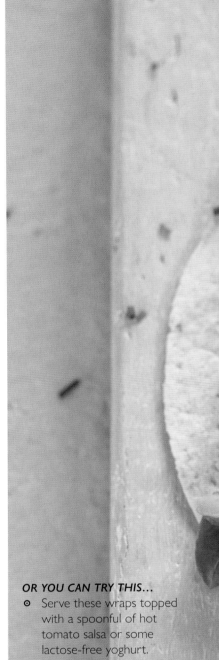

OR YOU CAN TRY THIS...

- Serve these wraps topped with a spoonful of hot tomato salsa or some lactose-free yoghurt.

- Add some grilled (broiled) peppers, courgettes (zucchini) or mushrooms to the wraps.

- Instead of chia, try adding fennel or cumin seeds.

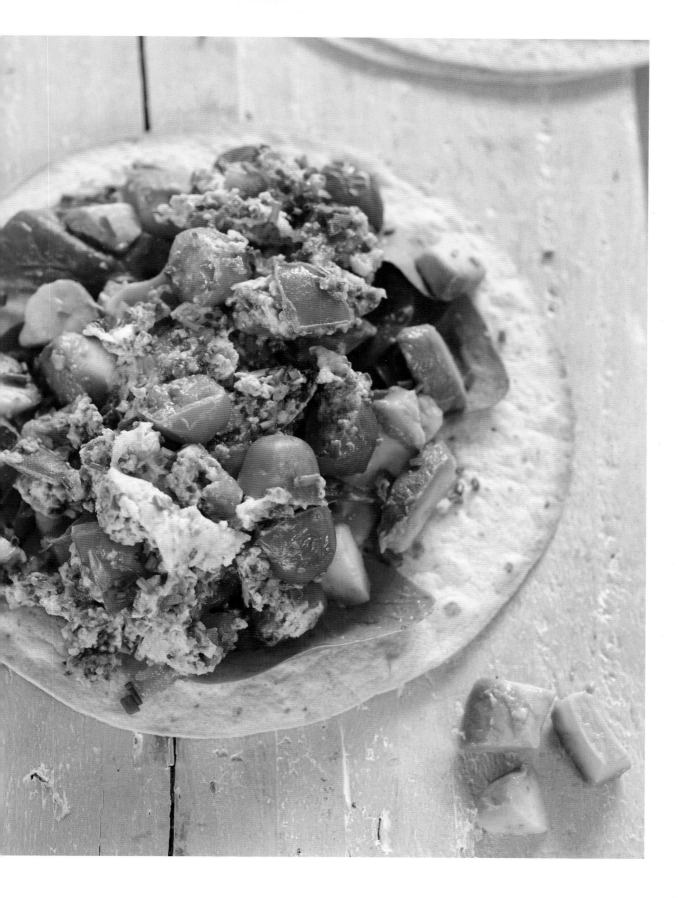

BUCKWHEAT PANCAKES
WITH BLUEBERRY COMPÔTE

You can use fresh or frozen blueberries to make the compôte – keep a packet in the freezer just in case. Or make double the quantity of batter and freeze the leftover pancakes between sheets of baking parchment to reheat for a quick breakfast or dessert.

MAKES 8 PANCAKES
PREP: 10 MIN
COOK: 20 MIN

250g/9oz (generous 2 cups) buckwheat flour

2 tsp baking powder

2 medium free-range eggs

250ml/9fl oz (1 generous cup) semi-skimmed milk or unsweetened almond milk, soy milk or lactose-free milk

1 tsp vanilla extract

1 tbsp maple syrup

2 tbsp melted butter

olive oil, for frying

4 heaped tbsp thick Greek yoghurt or lactose-free yoghurt

FOR THE BLUEBERRY COMPÔTE:

200g/7oz (2 cups) blueberries

60g/2oz (¼ cup) caster (superfine) sugar

a squeeze of lemon juice

1. Make the blueberry compôte: put two-thirds of the blueberries in a small pan with the sugar and 2 tablespoons water. Place over a low–medium heat and cook gently for 10 minutes, stirring until all the sugar has dissolved and the blueberries have burst. Add the remaining blueberries and cook for 5 minutes, until they soften but still retain their shape. Add a squeeze of lemon juice and set aside to cool a little.

2. Meanwhile, make the pancakes: sift the buckwheat flour and baking powder into a food processor. Add the eggs, and beat together. Add the milk, a little at a time, through the feed tube, beating all the time. Beat in the vanilla extract, maple syrup and melted butter until smooth. Alternatively, mix the batter in a bowl, using a hand whisk or hand-held electric whisk.

3. Heat a little olive oil in a large non-stick frying pan (skillet), swirling it around to lightly coat the bottom of the pan. Add 2–3 tablespoons of batter per pancake to the pan (you should be able to cook a couple of pancakes at a time in a large pan) and cook over a medium heat for 3–4 minutes until set and golden brown underneath. Flip the pancakes over and cook the other side. Remove and keep warm while you cook the remaining pancakes in the same way.

4. Serve the hot pancakes with the warm blueberry compôte and a spoonful of yoghurt.

OR YOU CAN TRY THIS...

- Instead of compôte, serve the pancakes with sliced banana, fresh strawberries or raspberries and lactose-free yoghurt, drizzled with maple syrup.

- Add a teaspoon of ground cinnamon or a good pinch of grated nutmeg to the batter for a subtle spicy flavour.

BREAKFAST BLT TOASTIE

A satisfying and tasty breakfast to start the day! This is a variation on the trend for avocado toast, transforming it into a more familiar sandwich.

SERVES 4
PREP: 5 MIN
COOK: 5 MIN

1 tbsp olive oil

8 baby plum tomatoes, halved

8 rashers (slices) lean back bacon

8 slices gluten-free bread

1 small ripe avocado, halved, peeled, stoned (pitted) and mashed

4 tsp mayonnaise

shredded iceberg lettuce

salt and freshly ground black pepper

1. Heat the olive oil in a frying pan (skillet) over a medium heat and cook the tomatoes for 3–4 minutes to soften them – don't overcook or they will fall apart.

2. Grill (broil) the bacon until crisp and golden and transfer to kitchen paper (towels) to absorb any fat.

3. Toast the bread lightly and spread 4 slices with the mashed avocado. Season with salt and pepper, then arrange 4 tomato halves and 2 bacon rashers on top of each slice.

4. Spread the mayonnaise over the remaining slices of toast and add some iceberg lettuce. Place on top of the avocado, tomato and bacon slices and cut each sandwich in half or into quarters. Eat immediately while still hot.

OR YOU CAN TRY THIS...

- Use any crisp lettuce leaves in these sandwiches.

- If you like really crisp bacon, try pancetta or thin-cut streaky bacon rashers.

- Flavour the mashed avocado with a dash of lemon or lime juice or some dried chilli (hot pepper) flakes.

- Add a dash of hot chilli sauce, harissa or Tabasco.

- Use toasted gluten-free English muffins instead of bread.

- Stuff the sandwich filling into split, warmed pittas or roll up in gluten-free wraps or cornmeal tortillas.

FULL ENGLISH TRAYBAKE BRUNCH

A full English is a great brunch for all the family at weekends, and the beauty of this recipe is that everything is cooked in a single roasting tray in the minimum of oil, making it really healthy.

SERVES 4
PREP: 10 MIN
COOK: 20–25 MIN

300g/10½oz baby spinach leaves

1 tbsp olive oil

8 small field or Portobello mushrooms

8 small tomatoes, halved

4 medium free-range eggs

2 tbsp grated Cheddar cheese (optional)

8 thin rashers (slices) lean smoked back bacon

a pinch of paprika or cayenne pepper

salt and freshly ground black pepper

1. Preheat the oven to 190°C, 375°F, gas mark 5.

2. Put the spinach in a colander and pour over freshly boiled water – it will wilt and turn bright green. Drain well, pressing out any excess water with a small plate or saucer.

3. Heat the oil in a large shallow roasting tin (pan) over a medium to high heat. Add the mushrooms, cook for 3–4 minutes and remove from the heat. Add the tomatoes, cut-side up, to the pan and bake in the preheated oven for 10 minutes.

4. Add the spinach, placing it in little heaps around the mushrooms and tomatoes. Make 4 indentations and break an egg into each one. Sprinkle lightly with the cheese (if using) and season with salt and pepper. Bake in the oven for 6–8 minutes until the eggs are set and the cheese melts.

5. Meanwhile, grill or dry-fry the bacon until golden brown and crisp. Crumble or chop into small pieces.

6. Sprinkle the bacon over the traybake and lightly dust with paprika or cayenne pepper. Serve immediately.

OR YOU CAN TRY THIS...

- If you can get gluten-free sausages without added onion or garlic, add them to the traybake.

- Use pancetta or very thinly sliced Parma ham instead of bacon.

- For a more substantial brunch or even supper, add some cubed new potatoes. Cook them in the oil for 5 minutes before adding the mushrooms.

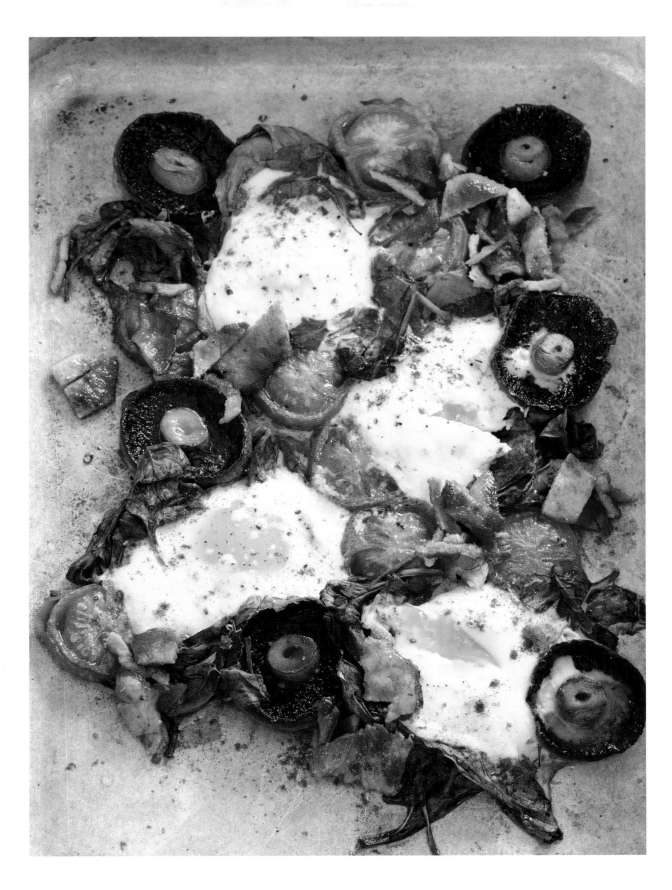

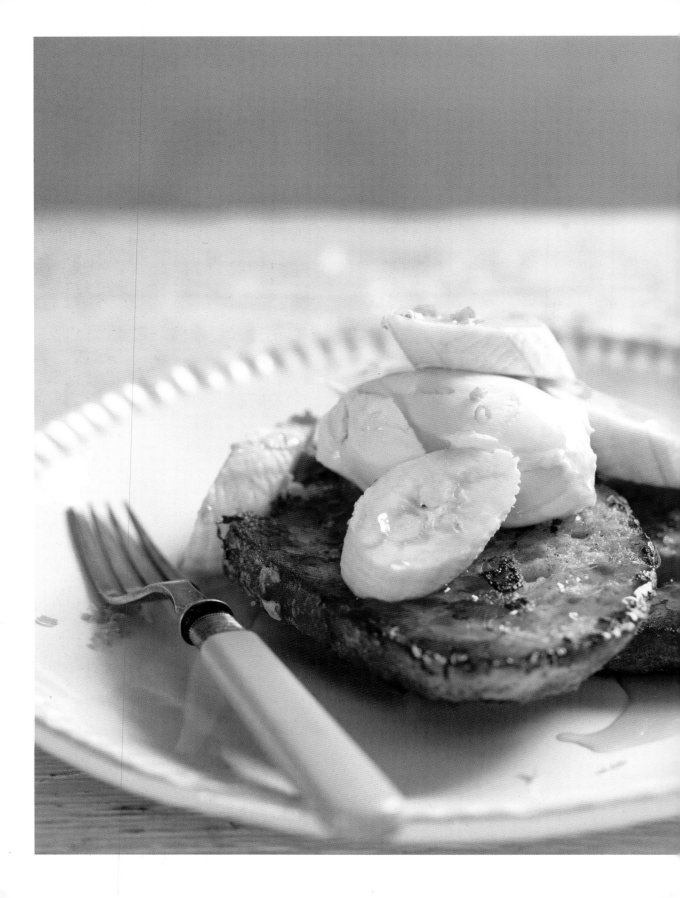

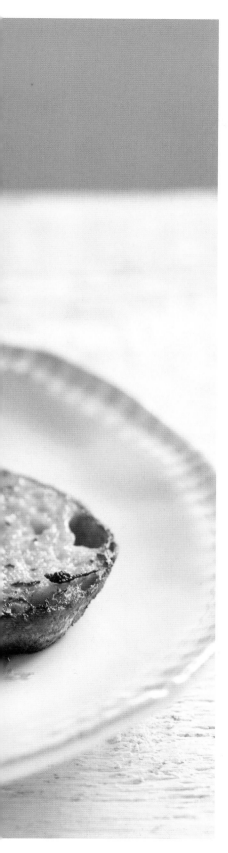

CINNAMON FRENCH TOAST
WITH CREAM CHEESE & BANANA

This is a delicious way of using up bread that is going stale and past its best. You can make it sweeter and even eat it as a dessert by dusting with icing (confectioner's) sugar. Using lactose-free cream cheese (keeps it FODMAP friendly.

SERVES 4
PREP: 10 MIN
COOK: 5 MIN

2 large free-range eggs

120ml/4fl oz (½ cup) milk or soya milk or lactose-free milk

a few drops of vanilla extract

½ tsp ground cinnamon

a pinch of freshly grated orground nutmeg

a pinch of salt

4 thick slices gluten-free bread

unsalted butter, for frying

freshly ground black pepper

4 tbsp lactose-free cream cheese

grated zest of 1 small orange

2 bananas, sliced

maple syrup, for drizzling

○ ○ ○

CINNAMON FRENCH TOAST

1. Beat the eggs with the milk, vanilla, spices and salt. Pour the mixture into a shallow dish.

2. Dip the slices of bread into the egg mixture and leave just long enough for the batter to penetrate the bread (usually less than 1 minute or 30 seconds each side) but not so long that the bread gets soggy and falls apart.

3. Heat the butter in a large frying pan (skillet) set over a medium heat. Add the soaked bread to the hot pan (do this in batches if necessary) and cook for 2–3 minutes until golden brown and crisp underneath. Turn the slices over and cook the other side.

4. Serve the French toast with a grinding of black pepper topped with a spoonful of cream cheese. Sprinkle with the orange zest. Add the sliced bananas and drizzle with maple syrup.

OR YOU CAN TRY THIS...

- Serve with fresh berries, such as strawberries, raspberries and blueberries, or make them into a compôte.

- Sprinkle the cooked French toast with ground spices instead of adding them to the batter.

- Vary the spices with ground ginger, mace or cloves.

- Use vegetable oil instead of butter to fry the French toast.

- If you can find them, gluten-free brioche and panettone work really well and elevate this dish into something truly special.

BAKED SPINACH & TOMATO EGGS

This makes a healthy brunch and it's so easy to prepare and cook. If you're in a hurry, you can speed it up by using frozen spinach instead of fresh.

SERVES 4
PREP: 10 MIN
COOK: 15–18 MIN

900g/2lb spinach, washed and trimmed

a pinch of grated nutmeg

1 tbsp olive oil

250g/9oz baby plum tomatoes, halved

4 medium free-range eggs

2 tbsp low-fat plain yoghurt or lactose-free yoghurt

a handful of dill, roughly chopped

salt and freshly ground black pepper

1. Preheat the oven to 180°C, 350°F, gas mark 4.

2. Put the damp spinach in a large saucepan over a medium heat, cover and cook for 1–2 minutes, shaking the pan occasionally, until the spinach wilts and turns bright green. Alternatively, pour some boiling water over the spinach in a colander or wilt in the microwave. Drain well, pressing out any excess water. Pat dry with kitchen paper (towels) and chop. Season with nutmeg, salt and pepper.

3. Heat the oil in a flameproof casserole dish, set over a low to medium heat. Add the tomatoes and cook for 2–3 minutes, then stir in the spinach and cook for 2 minutes. Remove from the heat and make 4 hollows in the spinach. Break an egg into each one.

4. Bake in the preheated oven for 10 minutes until the eggs are set. Spoon the yoghurt over the top and sprinkle with plenty of dill.

5. Serve immediately with toast or crusty bread.

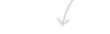

OR YOU CAN TRY THIS…

- Instead of baking in the oven, cook the tomatoes and spinach in a large deep frying pan, then add the eggs, cover the pan with a lid and set over a very low heat for at least 5 minutes until the eggs set.

- Add some diced mozzarella before baking. It will melt into the spinach and eggs.

- If your guests are hungry, use a bigger pan and two eggs per person.

EGG & BACON BREAKFAST SALAD

This salad is an unusual and healthy twist on the traditional eggs and bacon breakfast. You can serve it as a light lunch or supper, too.

SERVES 4
PREP: 10 MIN
COOK: 6–8 MIN

8 rashers (slices) lean back bacon

4 medium free-range eggs

1 tsp white wine vinegar

100g/3½oz mixed salad leaves

12 baby plum tomatoes, halved or quartered

2 tbsp vinaigrette dressing

balsamic vinegar, for drizzling

salt and freshly ground black pepper

snipped chives, for sprinkling

gluten-free bread, to serve

1. Grill (broil) or dry-fry the bacon until crisp and golden. Drain on kitchen paper (towels) to absorb any excess fat.

2. Poach the eggs with the vinegar in a pan of gently simmering water over a low heat for 3–4 minutes. When the whites are set but the yolks are still runny, remove with a slotted spoon.

3. Meanwhile, gently toss the salad leaves and tomatoes in the vinaigrette dressing. Divide between 4 serving plates and drizzle with balsamic vinegar.

4. Crumble or chop the bacon and scatter over the salad. Top each portion with a poached egg and season lightly with salt and pepper. Sprinkle with the chives and serve immediately with crusty bread.

OR YOU CAN TRY THIS...

⊙ Instead of mixed salad leaves and tomatoes, use baby spinach leaves and sliced grilled mushrooms.

⊙ Streaky bacon, pancetta or even diced ham can be added to the salad.

⊙ Toast the bread and brush with fruity olive oil. Break into small pieces and scatter over the salad.

ANYTHING-GOES FRITTATA

Frittatas are a brilliant way to use up whatever bits and bobs you have hanging around in the back of the fridge – anything really does go! If you're looking for a basic formula for a really satisfying start to the day, go for a couple of different types of vegetables (preferably one that's green), a bit of protein – although you will get some from the egg – a herb or a spice for a flavour boost, and some sort of cheese to melt over the top. See suggestions in the ingredients list, go for the combos listed below, or improvise entirely with what you have.

SERVES 4
PREP: 10 MIN
COOK: 18 MIN

1 tbsp olive oil (garlic infused, if you prefer)

8 medium free-range eggs

a selection of fillings, such as:
  wilted spinach, kale or chard leaves; a more substantial vegetable, such as roasted squash, aubergine (eggplant), (bell) peppers, courgettes (zucchini); shredded cooked meat or fish; herbs, such as tarragon, mint, parsley, basil, dill, etc; spices such as ground cumin and coriander, chilli powder or smoked paprika; grated cheese, such as Cheddar, goat's cheese, feta, Swiss, Parmesan

salt and freshly ground black pepper

1. Preheat the grill to high.

2. Whisk together the eggs in a jug, and season really well with salt and pepper. Stir in any vegetables, meat or fish, herbs, spices, and most of the cheese.

3. Lightly grease a 23cm/9in frying pan with a heatproof handle with a little olive oil and heat it over a low to medium heat. Pour in the egg mixture and cover the pan with a lid. Cook for about 10–15 minutes, until the mixture is firm on the bottom, but still slightly runny on the top.

4. Sprinkle the reserved cheese over the top of the frittata and place under the grill for a couple of minutes until the top is golden and bubbling and the frittata is cooked through. Transfer to a plate and cut into wedges to serve.

OR YOU CAN TRY THIS...
- Wilt chopped curly kale in a frying pan with a little butter and some sage. Stir this into the egg mixture with blue cheese and chunks of roasted squash.

- Go Asian, adding sliced spring onion (scallion) greens, slightly steamed pak choi (bok choy), a handful of bean sprouts, sliced red chilli and plenty of coriander (cilantro). Serve with slices of lime and soy sauce.

SNACKS

AMERICAN-STYLE STEAK SANDWICHES

A traditional steak sandwich is made with fried onions and possibly mushrooms, too, making it a 'no go' area on FODMAP. But you needn't miss out as this version is equally delicious and easy to make.

SERVES 4
PREP: 10 MIN
COOK: 10–14 MIN

olive oil, for brushing

2 red, green or yellow (bell) peppers, deseeded and sliced

4 thin lean sirloin or rump steaks, visible fat removed

8 slices gluten-free bread

4 tbsp mustard mayonnaise

4 slices Cheddar or Swiss cheese

salt and freshly ground black pepper

1. Brush a griddle pan with olive oil and place over a medium heat. Add the pepper strips and cook, turning occasionally, for about 5 minutes until tender and the edges are slightly charred. Remove and keep warm.

2. Cook the steaks in a lightly oiled frying pan (skillet) or on a griddle pan or under a hot grill (broiler) until done to your liking. Cooking times will vary depending on the type and thickness of the steaks, but as a general guide: 1½ minutes each side for rare; just over 2 minutes each side for medium; and 3 minutes each side for medium to well done.

3. Lightly toast the bread and spread 4 slices with the mayonnaise. Cut the steaks into thin slices and arrange on top. Cover with the cheese slices and pop under a preheated hot grill (broiler) for 1 minute until melted.

4. Spoon the warm peppers over the melted cheese and top with the remaining slices of toast. Cut the sandwiches in half and enjoy while they're still hot.

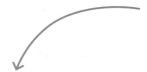

OR YOU CAN TRY THIS...

- Use regular mayonnaise and add some hot English or Dijon mustard.

- Omit the mustard and use horseradish instead.

- Try blue cheese, mozzarella or goat's cheese.

- Stir some chopped capers or dill pickles into the mayonnaise.

- If you're in a hurry, substitute bottled peppers.

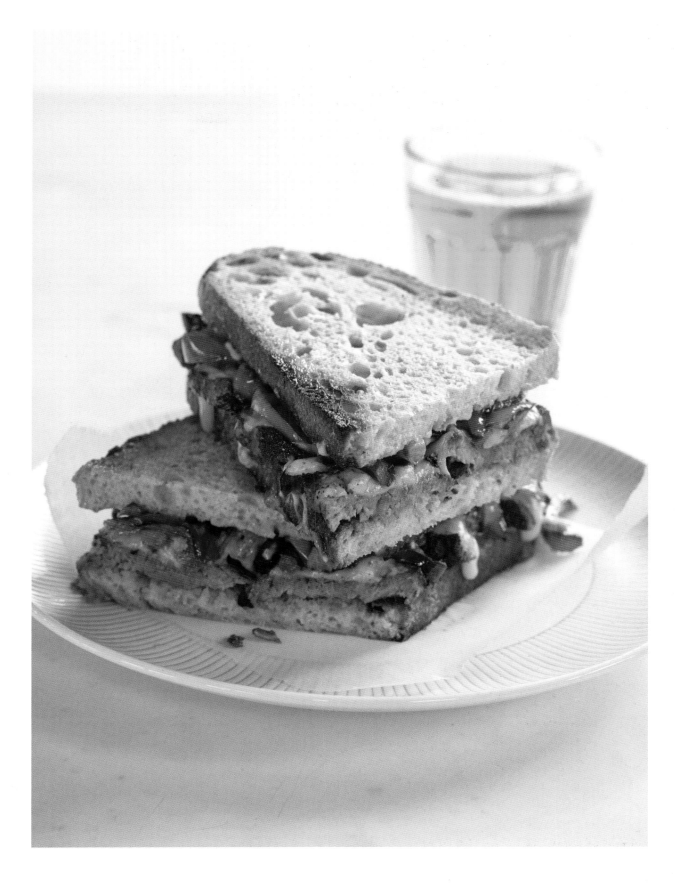

FRUITY TURKEY OPEN SANDWICH

Open sandwiches are easy to make for a quick snack or light lunch. Unless the bread is really fresh and delicious, it's best to toast it lightly – it will hold its shape better, too.

SERVES 4
PREP: 10 MIN

4 tbsp mayonnaise

1 small red chilli, deseeded and diced

2 tsp spicy mango chutney

225g/8oz cooked turkey breast, cubed

1 small mango, peeled, stoned (pitted) and diced

4 slices gluten-free bread, toasted if wished

4 tsp seeds, e.g. pumpkin, cumin or fennel

4 tsp chopped peanuts or hazelnuts

a handful of chives, snipped

salt and freshly ground black pepper

1. In a small bowl, mix the mayonnaise with the chilli, chutney, turkey and mango. Season to taste with salt and pepper.

2. Top the slices of bread with the turkey and fruit mixture, spreading it out evenly right up to the corners.

3. Scatter the seeds and nuts over the top and sprinkle with the chives.

OR YOU CAN TRY THIS...

- Substitute chicken, ham or prawns (shrimp) for the turkey.

- Use the turkey and fruit topping as a filling for sandwiches, cornmeal wraps or split warmed gluten-free pittas.

- Use diced papaya (pawpaw) instead of mango.

- Grill (broil) fresh chicken breasts and instead of adding it cold to the fruity mayonnaise, cut it into thin slices and arrange on top.

- Use toasted pine nuts instead of chopped nuts.

- Stir a tablespoon of dried cranberries or raisins into the filling.

- For a lighter filling, substitute thick Greek yoghurt for the mayonnaise.

CHICKEN & CHEDDAR QUESADILLAS

Quesadillas are much easier to make than they look. They are very versatile and you can add almost anything to the filling. Look at your list of FODMAP-friendly food and have fun experimenting with different flavours.

SERVES 4
PREP: 10 MIN
COOK: 8–12 MIN

110g/4oz (generous 1 cup) grated Cheddar cheese

225g/8oz cooked chicken breast fillets, shredded or chopped

1 red chilli, deseeded and diced

2 bottled roasted red (bell) peppers, chopped

a handful of coriander (cilantro), chopped

4 large cornmeal tortillas

olive oil, for brushing

salt and freshly ground black pepper

1. Mix together the grated cheese, chicken, chilli, peppers and coriander in a bowl. Season lightly with salt and pepper.

2. Set a large non-stick frying pan (skillet) over a medium heat. Lightly brush one of the tortillas with oil and place, oiled side down, in the hot pan. Spread half of the chicken and Cheddar mixture over the top leaving a thin border around the edge. Cover with another tortilla, pressing down gently to flatten it and around the edges to seal.

3. Cook for 2–3 minutes until the bottom tortilla is golden brown underneath. Use a spatula to turn the quesadilla over carefully and cook the other side. It's cooked when the underside is lightly browned and crisp and the cheese melts. Remove from the pan and keep warm while you cook the remaining tortillas and filling in the same way.

4. Cut each hot quesadilla into 6 triangles and serve immediately.

OR YOU CAN TRY THIS...

- Vegetarians can leave out the chicken and add a little diced avocado and tomato instead.

- Serve the quesadillas with lactose-free yoghurt.

- Instead of sandwiching the filling between 2 tortillas, cover half of each tortilla with the chicken and Cheddar mixture, then fold over and cook on both sides. Serve cut into 3 wedges.

- Use diced mozzarella or grated Monterey Jack cheese instead of Cheddar.

TANDOORI CHICKEN WRAPS

You can enjoy these wraps as a snack or serve them with boiled rice and a salad as a main course. Make sure you use cornmeal or gluten-free wraps – most supermarkets sell them.

SERVES 4
PREP: 15 MIN, PLUS CHILLING
COOK: 10–15 MIN

2 tbsp tandoori paste

juice of ½ lemon or lime

a good pinch of ground turmeric

180g/6oz (¾ cup) low-fat natural yoghurt or lactose-free yoghurt

400g/14oz skinned chicken breast fillets, cubed

4 large cornmeal tortilla wraps

crisp salad leaves

FOR THE CUCUMBER RAITA:
180g/6oz (¾ cup) low-fat yoghurt or lactose-free yoghurt

½ cucumber, diced

1 small bunch of mint or coriander (cilantro), chopped

a squeeze of lemon juice

1 tsp black mustard seeds

salt and freshly ground black pepper

1. Mix the tandoori paste, lemon or lime juice and turmeric with the yoghurt in a bowl. Add the chicken, turning it in the mixture until thoroughly coated. Cover and chill in the fridge for at least 30 minutes.

2. Meanwhile, make the cucumber raita: mix the yoghurt with the cucumber, chopped herbs and lemon juice. Season to taste with salt and pepper. Dry-fry the mustard seeds in a small frying pan (skillet) set over a high heat for 1–2 minutes, shaking the pan gently until the seeds pop and release their aroma. Remove from the pan and stir into the raita.

3. Put the tandoori-coated chicken on a foil-lined grill (broiler) pan and cook, turning occasionally, for 10–15 minutes until cooked right through and golden brown. Alternatively, cook in a lightly oiled griddle pan over a medium to high heat.

4. Warm the wraps in a low oven or on a griddle pan and divide the salad leaves and tandoori chicken between them. Spoon the raita over the top and fold over or roll up.

OR YOU CAN TRY THIS...

⊙ Instead of making the raita, top with some plain yoghurt or lactose-free yoghurt and onion- and garlic-free Indian pickle or chutney.

⊙ Or just drizzle with plain yoghurt or lactose-free yoghurt and sweet chilli sauce instead of raita.

⊙ Use turkey or even prawns (shrimp) instead of chicken.

BROWN RICE & TUNA SALAD
WITH JAPANESE DRESSING

You can buy packs of sprouted seeds in many supermarkets as well as health food stores, or you can sprout them yourself at home. They are a nutritional powerhouse, rich in vitamins and minerals.

SERVES 4
PREP: 15 MIN
COOK: 20 MIN

225g/8oz (1 cup) brown rice (dry weight)

150g/5oz (2¼ cups) sprouted seeds, e.g. alfalfa

2 tbsp black or white sesame seeds

olive oil, for brushing

4 x 125g/4oz tuna steaks

FOR THE JAPANESE DRESSING:
2 tbsp sunflower oil

1 tbsp toasted sesame oil

1 tbsp miso paste

1 tbsp rice vinegar or mirin

1 tbsp soy sauce

juice of ½ lime

2 tsp grated fresh root ginger

1 tsp sugar

1. Cook the brown rice according to the instructions on the packet. Remove from the pan and leave to cool in a large bowl.

2. Make the Japanese dressing: whisk all the ingredients together until well mixed or place in a screwtop jar and shake vigorously.

3. Gently stir the rice with a fork to separate the grains. Mix in the sprouted seeds and pour most of the dressing over the top. Toss gently together.

4. Dry-fry the sesame seeds in a small frying pan (skillet) set over a medium to high heat for 1–2 minutes until they release their aroma. Make sure they don't burn. Remove from the pan and set aside to cool.

5. Lightly oil a non-stick griddle pan and place over a medium to high heat. Add the tuna steaks to the hot pan and cook for 2–3 minutes on each side, depending on how well cooked you like them. Cut each steak into slices.

6. Put a mound of rice salad on each serving plate and top with the sliced tuna. Drizzle with the remaining dressing and sprinkle with the toasted sesame seeds.

OR YOU CAN TRY THIS...

- Use griddled salmon, chicken, steak or tofu instead of tuna.

- Serve the tuna and rice with some steamed green beans or pak choi (bok choy).

- Rice or soba noodles tossed in the dressing make a tasty alternative to brown rice.

VIETNAMESE SHRIMP SPRING ROLLS

You will need a pack of translucent rice paper wrappers to make these crunchy snacks – you can buy them online or from Asian stores and some supermarkets. These spring rolls are healthier and lower in calories than traditional deep-fried ones.

SERVES 4
PREP: 15 MIN
COOK: 5 MIN

1 tbsp sunflower or groundnut (peanut) oil
1 red (bell) pepper, deseeded and diced
100g/3½oz carrots, cut into thin matchsticks
85g/3oz spring greens or kale, shredded
60g/2oz (½ cup) bean sprouts
150g/5oz cooked peeled prawns (shrimp)
2 tbsp soy sauce
3 tbsp chopped coriander (cilantro)
4 gluten-free rice paper (spring roll) wrappers
sweet chili sauce, for dipping

1. Heat the oil in a wok or large frying pan (skillet) set over a high heat and stir-fry the pepper and carrots for 2 minutes. Add the spring greens, bean sprouts and prawns and stir-fry for 2 minutes. Stir in the soy sauce and coriander and remove from the heat.

2. Dip a rice paper wrapper into a bowl of cold water – just long enough for it to become softened and pliable.

3. Lay softened wrapper out flat on a clean work surface or board and place one-quarter of the vegetable and prawn mixture in the centre. Fold the sides over the filling to enclose it and roll up tightly like a parcel.

4. Repeat this process with the remaining rice wrappers and filling, so you have 4 spring rolls.

5. Serve the spring rolls immediately with chilli sauce for dipping. Or you can eat them cold if preferred.

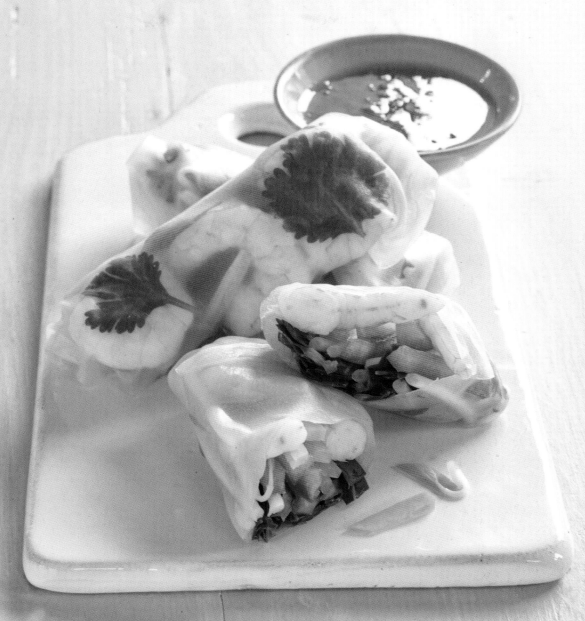

OR YOU CAN TRY THIS...

- Use cooked diced chicken instead of shrimp.

- Leave out the shrimp and make a veggie version, adding some yellow (bell) pepper or courgette (zucchini).

DELI VEGETABLE ROLL UPS

Sweet roasted veggies with a light cheese filling make great healthy snacks to have on hand. If you want to make them into a more substantial lunch, add cooked rice, quinoa or buckwheat to the filling.

SERVES 4–6
PREP: 20 MIN
COOK: 10–20 MIN

2 red or yellow (bell) peppers

1 large aubergine (eggplant)

2 large courgettes (zucchini)

olive oil, for brushing

FOR THE COTTAGE CHEESE FILLING:
110g/4oz (generous ½ cup) plain cottage cheese or lactose-free cottage cheese

1 tomato, diced

a few chives, snipped

salt and freshly ground black pepper

FOR THE SPINACH AND CREAM CHEESE FILLING:
110g/4oz baby spinach leaves

60g/2oz (¼ cup) light cream cheese or lactose-free cream cheese

2 tbsp light mayonnaise

a few sprigs of dill, chopped

1. Place the peppers under a preheated hot grill (broiler), turning occasionally, until the skins blister and start to char. Remove and pop them into a plastic bag. When they are cool enough to handle, remove from the bag, peel off the skins and cut them in half. Discard the cores and seeds. Trim the pepper halves so you end up with 8 rectangles. Don't waste the trimmings — dice them and set aside.

2. Meanwhile, slice the aubergine and courgettes lengthways into long thin strips. Cook in batches in an oiled griddle pan over a medium heat for about 5 minutes, turning them once, until just tender and golden brown on both sides. Remove carefully and set aside while you cook the remaining strips.

3. Make the cottage cheese filling: mix the cottage cheese with the tomato and chives. Add the reserved grilled (broiled) pepper trimmings and season with salt and pepper.

4. Make the spinach and cream cheese filling: put the spinach in a colander and pour over freshly boiled water. It will wilt and turn bright green. Press down with a saucer to extract all the moisture and then pat dry with kitchen paper (towels). Chop and mix with the remaining ingredients, and season.

5. Divide the fillings between the griddled aubergine and courgette strips and the pepper rectangles. Roll them up like Swiss rolls (jelly rolls) around the filling. Wrap in cling film (plastic wrap) and chill until required.

OR YOU CAN TRY THIS...

- ◉ Make the fillings in advance and keep in airtight containers in the fridge.

- ◉ Fill with cooked quinoa or rice flavoured with herbs, spices, chilli or a dash of pesto, harissa or chilli sauce.

DOLMADES
WITH LEMON SAUCE (AVGOLEMONO)

These tender little bundles can be eaten as a snack, an appetizer, part of a *meze* or with pre-dinner drinks. You can buy packets or jars of vine leaves preserved in brine from delicatessens and many supermarkets. If you have a vine or can get the real thing, wash the fresh leaves and blanch them in boiling water, then drain and cool in a colander before filling and cooking as outlined below.

MAKES 24 DOLMADES
PREP: 20 MIN
COOK: 1 HOUR

24 vine leaves, preserved in brine

110g/4oz (generous ½ cup)
    basmati rice (dry weight)

2 tomatoes, diced

1 small bunch of dill, finely
    chopped

a handful of parsley, finely chopped

30g/1oz (generous ¼ cup) pine nuts

a good pinch of ground cumin

grated zest and juice of 1 lemon

about 600ml/1 pint (2½ cups)
    onion-free chicken stock

salt and freshly ground black pepper

FOR THE LEMON SAUCE:
2 medium free-range eggs

4 tbsp lemon juice

stock from cooking dolmades
    (above)

OR YOU CAN TRY THIS…

- Instead of making the lemon sauce, serve the dolmades cold with a bowl of lactose-free yoghurt or tzatziki.

- You can add raisins, sultanas (golden raisins) or currants to the rice filling.

1. Rinse the vine leaves and remove the stems. Drain in a colander.

2. Make the stuffing: cook the rice according to the instructions on the packet. Fluff up the rice to separate the grains and mix with the tomatoes, herbs, pine nuts, cumin and lemon zest. Season to taste with salt and pepper

3. Divide the stuffing between the vine leaves, placing a little on each one and then rolling up the leaf around it and tucking in the ends to seal securely.

4. Arrange the stuffed leaves, seam-side down, in the bottom of a saucepan, packing them in tightly. You can add another layer of dolmades on top if the pan is not large enough to hold them all in a single layer. Pour over enough hot stock to just cover them and add the lemon juice. Weight the dolmades down with a plate.

5. Cover the pan with a lid and simmer gently over a low heat for at least 45 minutes until the dolmades are tender and plump, checking them occasionally to make sure there's enough stock and adding more as needed. Lift them out carefully and transfer to a warm serving dish while you make the sauce. Reserve the cooking stock.

6. Beat the eggs in a bowl and then whisk in the lemon juice. Strain the reserved stock into a measuring jug and pour 300ml/10fl oz (1¼ cups) of it into a saucepan (add some water if you don't have enough). Bring to the boil and then whisk some of it into the eggs.

7. Tip the egg mixture into the stock in the pan and keep stirring with a wooden spoon over a low heat until the sauce thickens — do not let it boil or it will separate. Pour over the dolmades and serve immediately.

STICKY BUFFALO WINGS

These crisp aromatic chicken wings make delicious snacks. Check the labels carefully on the sauces you use – some are not low-FODMAP. Look for gluten-free, sucrose-free and garlic-free brands. Here they are used in very small quantities but you can make your own FODMAP-friendly ketchup and chilli sauce if you use them often.

SERVES 4
PREP: 10 MIN
CHILL: 30 MIN
COOK: 10–15 MIN

1 tbsp gluten-free
    hoisin sauce

2 tbsp reduced-sugar
    tomato ketchup
    (onion- and garlic-free)

1 tbsp dark soy sauce

1 tbsp sweet chilli sauce
    (garlic-free)

grated zest and juice of
    1 orange

12 chicken wings, cut
    in half

freshly ground black
    pepper

FOR LEMONY HERB DIP:
180g/6oz (scant 1 cup)
    0% fat Greek yoghurt
    or lactose-free yoghurt

a few fresh chives, snipped

grated zest of 1 lemon

a handful of coriander
    (cilantro) or parsley,
    finely chopped

1. Make the lemony herb dip: mix all the ingredients together in a bowl. Cover and leave to chill in the fridge.

2. Mix the hoisin sauce, ketchup, soy and chilli sauces, orange zest and juice together in a bowl. Add a good grinding of black pepper.

3. Add the halved chicken wings and turn them in the marinade until they are coated all over. Cover with cling film (plastic wrap) and leave to chill in the fridge for at least 30 minutes.

4. Preheat the grill (broiler). Remove the chicken wings from the marinade and place them on a foil-lined grill (broiler) tray. Spoon any remaining marinade over the top, then cook under the hot grill for 10–15 minutes, turning occasionally and basting with the marinade until really crisp and cooked through.

5. Serve the hot buffalo wings immediately with the lemony herb dip.

PORK WONTONS

These are coated in rice vermicelli, which pops up when fried, creating spiky, fun-looking balls. Some vermicelli noodle brands work better than others, so it's worth experimenting. Serve as cocktail nibbles or as a prelude to a stir-fried main course, accompanied by a soy sauce dip, flavoured with chopped chilli and sesame oil, if you like.

SERVES 4
PREP: 10 MIN
COOK: 12 MIN

2.5cm/1in piece fresh root ginger, peeled and roughly chopped

1 tbsp lemongrass paste

2 hot chillies (deseed for a milder heat)

1 tsp salt

2 tsp Thai fish sauce (nam pla)

grated zest and juice of 1 lime

a small bunch of fresh coriander (cilantro), roughly chopped

450g/1lb (2 cups) minced (ground) pork

3–4 nests of white rice vermicelli noodles (dry weight)

2 eggs, beaten

white rice flour, for coating

sunflower or vegetable oil, for deep-frying

salt and freshly ground black pepper

sweet chilli sauce, to serve

1. Put the ginger, lemongrass paste, chillies and salt in the small bowl of a food processor and process until finely chopped. Add the fish sauce, lime zest and juice and coriander and pulse again to just combine.

2. Put the pork in a large bowl and add the spice paste. Mix until well combined. If you want to check the seasoning, fry off a little bit of the mixture to taste it.

3. Crush the noodle nests with your hands to break the noodles into short lengths. Put them in a shallow bowl. Put the beaten eggs in another shallow bowl, and the rice flour into a third bowl.

4. Pour the oil for frying into a saucepan to a depth of about 5cm/2in. Heat it to 180°C/350°F. Use a thermometer to check this, as the right temperature is quite important – too cold and the noodles will not pop properly and be hard; too hot and they will burn before the pork balls cook all the way through.

5. Using floured hands, shape the pork mixture into walnut-sized balls, weighing around 30g/1oz each – you should make 16. Roll them first in the flour, then in the beaten egg, and then in the crushed noodles. Gently but firmly press the noodles into the balls as you coat them, then gently shake off any excess.

6. Deep-fry the balls, in batches of 4, for 2–3 minutes until golden brown on all sides and the pork is cooked right through. Get the oil back up to temparture in between each batch. Drain on crumpled kitchen paper. Serve warm with a sauce for dipping.

LOADED POTATO SKINS
WITH DIFFERENT TOPPINGS

These loaded potato skins make great snacks or you can even serve them for a light lunch or supper with salad. For parties, use really small potatoes and make mini ones.

SERVES 4 (4 POTATO SKINS EACH)
PREP: 15 MINS
COOK: 1–1¼ HOURS

8 small baking potatoes

olive oil, for rubbing

sea salt crystals

FOR THE CHEESE AND HAM TOPPING:
110g/4oz (generous ½ cup) grated Cheddar cheese

110g/4oz (scant 1 cup) cooked ham, diced

1–2 tsp Dijon mustard

a handful of chives, snipped

FOR THE PIZZA TOPPING:
1 tbsp garlic-infused olive oil

1 x 400g/14oz can chopped tomatoes

1–2 tbsp tomato paste

a pinch of sugar

a few sprigs of basil, chopped

a few drops of balsamic vinegar

110g/4oz (1 cup) diced mozzarella cheese

salt and freshly ground black pepper

1. Preheat the oven to 200°C, 400°F, gas mark 6.

2. Prick the potatoes all over with a fork. Put them in a baking dish and pour over a little olive oil. Rub it into the potato skins and then sprinkle with sea salt crystals. Bake in the preheated oven for 45–60 minutes until the skins are crisp and the insides are soft and cooked. Remove and set aside until cool enough to handle.

3. Make the cheese and ham topping: mix all the ingredients together in a bowl and set aside.

4. Make the tomato sauce for the pizza topping: heat the oil in a frying pan (skillet) over a low to medium heat and add the tomatoes. Stir in the tomato paste, sugar and basil and cook for 8–10 minutes until the sauce is thick and reduced. Season with salt and pepper and a few drops of balsamic vinegar.

5. Split the potatoes in half lengthways and scoop out the insides. Mix half the scooped-out potato with the cheese and ham topping mixture, and the rest with the tomato sauce for the pizza topping..

6. Spoon each type of topping mixture into 8 potato skins. Sprinkle the diced mozzarella over the skins topped with the tomato and potato mixture. Placeall the topped potato skins under a preheated hot grill (broiler) until the cheese melts.

OR YOU CAN TRY THIS…

- Use crumbled crispy bacon bits instead of ham for the cheese and ham topping.

- Substitute grated Swiss cheese for Cheddar.

- Add some diced chilli or (bell) peppers to the tomato sauce.

- Sprinkle the loaded potato skins with chopped coriander (cilantro) before serving.

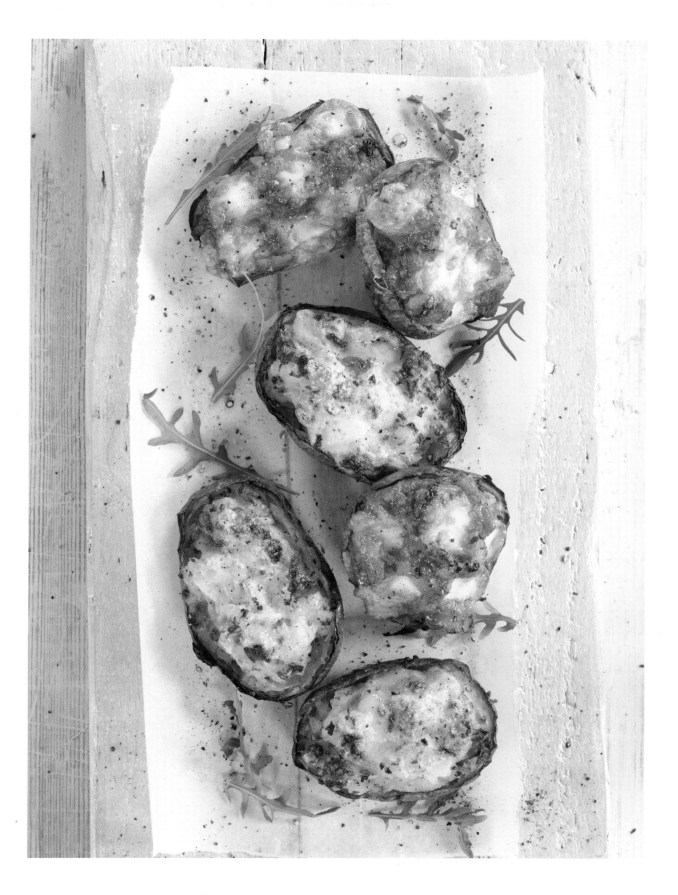

TOFU & VEGGIE SKEWERS

If you're not familiar with tofu, this easy snack is a delicious way to try it. Versatile, healthy and low in fat, tofu is a great source of vegetable protein. Made from bean curd, it has a pleasantly mild flavour and is a low-FODMAP food.

SERVES 4
PREP: 15 MIN
MARINATE: 15 MIN
COOK: 5–10 MIN

400g/14oz firm tofu, cubed

2 tbsp gluten-free and garlic-free teriyaki sauce

2 courgettes (zucchini), cut into chunks

1 red (bell) pepper, deseeded and cut into chunks

1 yellow (bell) pepper, deseeded and cut into chunks

1 small aubergine (eggplant), cut into chunks

olive oil

100g/3½oz wild rocket (arugula)

a few drops of balsamic vinegar

salt and freshly ground black pepper

4 tsp sweet chilli sauce, to serve

1. Put the tofu and teriyaki sauce in a bowl and stir gently. Leave to marinate in a cool place or the fridge for at least 15 minutes.

2. Thread the tofu cubes and courgettes, peppers and aubergine alternately onto 8 kebab skewers, brushing the vegetables with any leftover marinade.

3. Cook over hot coals on a barbecue or arrange the skewers in a foil-lined grill (broiler) pan and cook under a preheated hot grill (broiler) for 5–10 minutes, turning them occasionally, until the vegetables are tender and starting to char and the tofu is golden brown.

4. Serve immediately with some rocket drizzled with balsamic vinegar, with a teaspoon of chilli sauce on the side.

TIP
If you can't find a gluten-free and garlic-free teriyaki sauce, look for a soy sauce alternative.

MARINATED OLIVES & SPICED NUTS

Stuffed olives look great in this mixture, but make sure they are stuffed with pimiento peppers, or the like, rather than garlic cloves. Serve both mixes with drinks, or layer olives in small pots to use as gifts. It's best to prepare the olives in advance to allow them to fully absorb the flavours, while the nuts are great warm out of the oven and will go stale if stored for too long.

**MAKES 450G/1LB EACH
PREP: 20 MIN, PLUS
MARINATING (OLIVES)
COOK (NUTS): 30 MIN**

FOR THE OLIVES:

200g/7oz each black, green and stuffed olives

2 tbsp coriander seeds

finely grated zest of 1 orange, shredded

a few fresh coriander (cilantro) sprigs

480–750ml/16–26fl oz (2–3¼ cups) extra-virgin olive oil (depending on size of jar)

FOR THE NUTS:

350g/12oz mixed skinned nuts, such as almonds, pecans, hazelnuts

110g/4oz shelled mixed pumpkin and sunflower seeds

40g/1½oz (3 tbsp) butter or 3 tbsp sunflower oil

1 tbsp curry powder or garam masala

1 tsp coarse sea salt

1. Using a rolling pin, lightly hit each black and green olive to split without crushing completely. Alternatively, slit with a small sharp knife. (Stoned olives do not need cracking).

2. Arrange the black, green and stuffed olives in layers in an attractive 1.2 litre/40fl oz (5 cup) glass jar. Sprinkle each layer with coriander seeds and orange zest shreds. Tuck a few sprigs of coriander down the side of the jar.

3. Warm the olive oil in a saucepan to release the aroma, then pour sufficient into the jar to cover the olives completely. Tapping the jar to release any air bubbles, seal tightly and allow to cool. Leave in a cool dark place for 1 month to mature.

4. To prepare the nuts, preheat the oven to 150°C, 300°F, gas mark 2. Melt the butter in a roasting tin (pan), or pour sunflower oil into the roasting tin (pan) is using, and stir in the curry powder. Cook, stirring, for 30 seconds. Add the nuts and seeds and stir until well coated.

5. Roast nuts and seeds in the preheated oven for 30 minutes, stirring from time to time. On removing from the oven, immediately toss the nuts with the salt. Serve warm, or allow to cool completely and store for up to 2 weeks.

MEDITERRANEAN GRIDDLED VEGETABLE & FETA BRUSCHETTA

Bruschetta are great as a healthy snack, appetizer or even for party canapés. The thicker and crustier the bread the better.

SERVES 4
PREP: 15 MIN
COOK: 15 MIN

1–2 tbsp olive oil, plus extra for drizzling

1 red (bell) pepper, deseeded and cut into strips

1 yellow or green (bell) pepper, deseeded and cut into strips

1 small aubergine (eggplant), thinly sliced

2 courgettes (zucchini), thinly sliced or chopped

2 tsp capers

balsamic vinegar, for drizzling

4 thick slices gluten-free bread

4 tsp green pesto

110g/4oz feta cheese, crumbled

4 tbsp chopped herbs, e.g. thyme, basil or flat-leaf parsley

dried chilli (hot pepper) flakes, for sprinkling (optional)

salt and freshly ground black pepper

◦ ◦ ◦

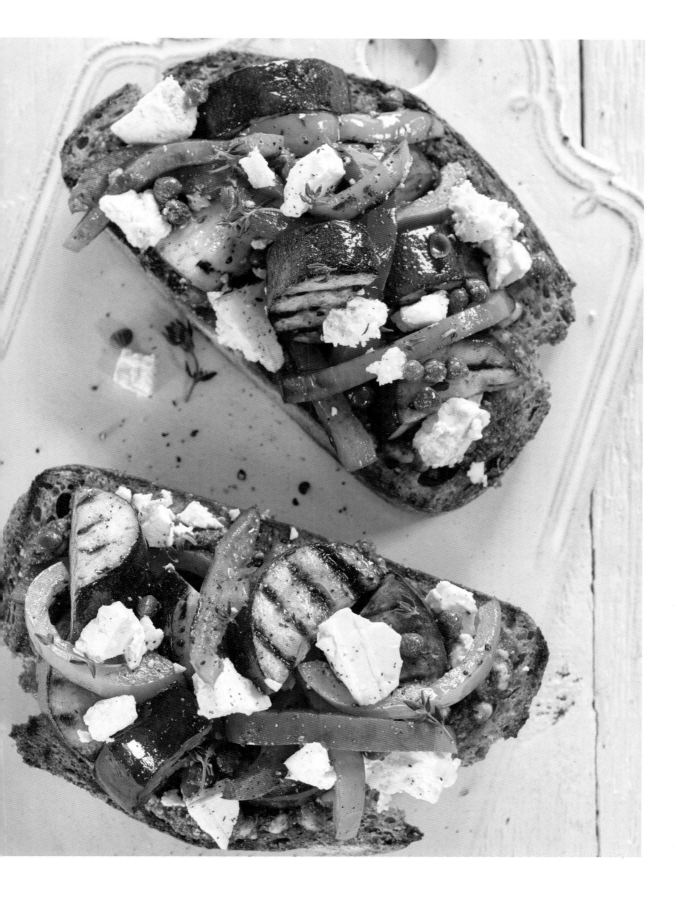

⚬⚬⚬ MEDITERRANEAN GRIDDLED VEGETABLE & FETA

1. Brush a griddle pan with the olive oil and set over a medium to high heat. Add half of the peppers, aubergine and courgettes to the hot pan and cook, turning occasionally, for about 5 minutes until just tender and starting to get charred around the edges. Remove and keep warm while you cook the rest of the vegetables in the same way.

2. Mix the griddled vegetables with the capers. Drizzle a little balsamic vinegar over the top, and season to taste.

3. Lightly toast the bread or place on the hot griddle for 1–2 minutes each side. Drizzle with olive oil and spread lightly with pesto.

4. Spoon the griddled vegetables over the top and add the crumbled feta. Sprinkle with herbs and chilli flakes (if using) and serve warm.

OR YOU CAN TRY THIS...

- ⊙ Instead of feta, sprinkle with grated Cheddar and pop under a hot grill (broiler) to melt.

- ⊙ Add sliced or diced mushrooms or fennel.

- ⊙ Instead of pesto, smear a little mashed avocado over the toast.

- ⊙ Use bottled precooked peppers and roasted vegetables.

- ⊙ Use garlic-infused olive oil.

POTATO & DILL PANCAKES
WITH SMOKED SALMON

These light potato pancakes, delicately flavoured with dill, melt in the mouth. They are simple to make and just need a slice of smoked salmon for a satisfying snack.

SERVES 4
PREP: 20 MIN
COOK: 25 MIN

250g/9oz floury potatoes

1 small egg

60ml/2fl oz (¼ cup) semi-skimmed milk, soya milk or lactose-free milk

2 tbsp white rice flour

½ tsp baking powder

a small handful of dill sprigs, roughly chopped, plus extra to serve

¼ tsp salt

30g/1oz (2 tbsp) unsalted butter, for frying

lemon wedges, to serve

thick Greek yogurt, to serve (optional)

1. Peel the potatoes and cut into evensized pieces. Cook in lightly salted boiling water for 12–15 minutes until tender. Drain well and mash until very smooth. Allow to cool slightly, then whisk in the egg, milk, flour, baking powder, dill and salt to form a thick smooth batter.

2. Preheat the oven to its lowest setting. Heat a tablespoon of butter in a non-stick frying pan set over a medium heat. Spoon in 2 large spoonfuls of the batter to form 2 pancakes and cook for about 2 minutes until golden. Flip the pancakes over and cook the other sides until golden brown and slightly risen. Keep warm in the oven. Repeat with the remaining mixture to make 4 pancakes in total.

3. Serve the pancakes with a slice of smoked salmon, a few sprigs of dill, a lemon wedge for squeezing and a spoonful of Greek yogurt, if you like.

OR YOU CAN TRY THIS...
- Switch the dill in the pancake for thyme and top with a fried egg.

SALADS

STEAK, ORANGE & BLUE CHEESE SALAD

If you remove all the visible fat from the steaks, this simple salad becomes a healthy light meal. Serve it with gluten-free bread to mop up any dressing and juices from the steak.

SERVES 4
PREP: 10 MIN
COOK: 8–11 MIN

1 tbsp olive oil

400g/14oz lean sirloin or fillet steaks, all visible fat removed

200g/7oz fine green beans, trimmed

2 juicy oranges, cut into segments

2 heads white or red chicory (Belgian endive), sliced

2 handfuls of rocket (arugula) or watercress

2 tbsp snipped chives or chopped tarragon

salt and freshly ground black pepper

FOR THE BLUE CHEESE DRESSING:
3 tbsp olive oil

1 tbsp red wine vinegar

juice of ½ lemon

60g/2oz creamy blue cheese, e.g. Danish Blue or gorgonzola, crumbled

1. Make the blue cheese dressing: whisk all the ingredients together until well blended.

2. Heat the olive oil in a frying pan (skillet) or griddle pan over a medium to high heat. Season the steaks and add to the pan. Cook them for 2–3 minutes each side for medium rare (longer if you like them well done). Remove and leave for 10 minutes before cutting them into slices.

3. Steam the green beans or cook in a pan of salted boiling water for 4–5 minutes until just tender but still a little crisp. Drain in a colander and cool under running cold water. Drain well and pat dry with kitchen paper (towels).

4. Toss the orange segments, chicory, rocket or watercress and green beans in most of the dressing. Divide between 4 serving plates, placing the steak strips on top. Drizzle with the remaining dressing and sprinkle with herbs.

OR YOU CAN TRY THIS...

- Use Dijon mustard instead of blue cheese in the dressing.

- Scatter some chopped walnuts over the salad.

- Make it more substantial by mixing in some cubes of roasted sweet potato (no more than 85g/3oz per serving).

WARM VIETNAMESE CHICKEN SALAD

You can make this salad more substantial and eat it for supper by mixing in some cooked thin rice noodles just before serving.

SERVES 4
PREP: 20 MIN
COOK: 8 MIN

½ cucumber, cut into very thin strips

2 carrots, cut into very thin strips

2 courgettes (zucchini), cut into thin strips

16 mangetout (snow pea) pods, trimmed and halved lengthways

110g/4oz beansprouts

2 Little Gem lettuces, leaves separated

2 tbsp groundnut (peanut) or olive oil

450g/1lb chicken breast fillets, cut into thin strips

a handful of mint, chopped

a handful of coriander (cilantro), chopped

2 tbsp coarsely chopped unsalted roasted peanuts

lime wedges, to serve

FOR THE VIETNAMESE DRESSING:
1 Thai red chilli, deseeded and shredded

2 tbsp fish sauce (nam pla)

1 tbsp light soy sauce

1 tbsp rice wine vinegar or water

juice of 1 lime

1 tsp sugar

freshly ground black pepper

1. Mix together the cucumber, carrots, courgettes, mangetout, beansprouts and lettuce in a large bowl.

2. Heat the oil in a non-stick griddle pan or frying pan (skillet) over a medium heat. Cook the chicken for about 6–8 minutes, turning occasionally, until cooked right through and golden brown.

3. Meanwhile, mix all the dressing ingredients together in a bowl or shake in a screwtop jar. Pour most of the dressing over the prepared vegetables in the bowl and toss to mix well.

4. Divide the vegetables between 4 serving plates. Top with the griddled warm chicken, then sprinkle with the herbs and peanuts. Drizzle the remaining dressing over the top and serve immediately with lime wedges.

OR YOU CAN TRY THIS...
- Substitute griddled turkey, steak or even prawns (shrimp) for the chicken.
- Use leftover cold roast chicken or turkey.

CHICKEN SATAY SALAD

Here the traditional Indonesian spicy chicken skewers and peanut sauce are transformed into a delicious salad.

SERVES 4
PREP: 20 MIN
COOK: 15 MIN

1–2 tbsp groundnut (peanut) oil or olive oil

400g/14oz boned chicken breasts

100g/3½oz rice noodles (dry weight)

1 carrot, cut into thin matchsticks

110g/4oz Chinese leaves (Chinese cabbage), shredded

1 red (bell) pepper, deseeded and cut into thin strips

1 yellow (bell) pepper, deseeded and cut into thin strips

85g/3oz radishes, thinly sliced

¼ cucumber, cut into matchsticks

a handful of fresh coriander (cilantro), chopped

2 tbsp roughly crushed salted roasted peanuts

seeds of ½ pomegranate

FOR THE SATAY DRESSING:
2 tbsp crunchy peanut butter

1 tbsp soy sauce

1 tbsp sweet chilli sauce

1 tsp groundnut (peanut) oil or sesame oil

juice of ½ lime

1 tsp caster (superfine) sugar

1. Heat the oil in a non-stick frying pan (skillet) or griddle pan over a medium heat. Cook the chicken for 12–15 minutes, turning halfway through, until cooked inside and golden brown. Cut into thin strips.

2. Mix the satay dressing ingredients in a bowl with 1 tablespoon water and add the warm chicken. Turn it over in the sauce until well coated.

3. Meanwhile, cook the rice noodles according to the directions on the packet. Drain well.

4. Put the chicken and noodles in a large bowl with the carrot, Chinese leaves, peppers, radishes, cucumber and coriander. Toss lightly together.

5. Divide the salad between 4 serving plates and sprinkle with the crushed peanuts and pomegranate seeds. Serve immediately.

OR YOU CAN TRY THIS...

- For a vegetarian option, use smoked tofu instead of chicken.

- If wished, you can warm the satay dressing ingredients in a small pan or in the microwave before using to coat the chicken.

- Prawns (shrimp) and turkey also work well.

WARM BUCKWHEAT & GOAT'S CHEESE SALAD

The sweet Thai-style dressing complements the earthy buckwheat, creamy goat's cheese and crunchy sprouts and green vegetables in this delicious salad.

SERVES 4
PREP: 15 MIN
COOK: 10 MIN

100g/3½oz (scant ¾ cup) roasted buckwheat (kasha)

200g/7oz fine green beans, trimmed and halved

100g/3½oz tenderstem broccoli, trimmed and each stalk cut in half

2 tbsp sesame seeds

85g/3oz (1½ cups) sun-blush tomatoes in olive oil

110g/4oz (2 cups) mixed sprouted seeds, e.g. alfalfa

1 small bunch of chives, snipped

150g/5oz soft creamy goat's cheese, cut into pieces

a pinch of dried chilli (hot pepper) flakes

salt and freshly ground black pepper

FOR THE SESAME VINAIGRETTE:
3 tbsp sunflower or groundnut (peanut) oil

1 tsp toasted sesame oil

1 tbsp light soy sauce

1 tbsp nam pla (Thai fish sauce)

juice of 1 lime

1 tsp grated fresh root ginger

1 tsp sugar

⊙ ⊙ ⊙

WARM BUCKWHEAT & GOAT'S CHEESE SALAD

1. Mix the vinaigrette ingredients together in a bowl or shake in a screwtop jar until thoroughly mixed.

2. Cook the buckwheat: bring 150ml/5fl oz (generous ½ cup) water to the boil in a saucepan. Reduce the heat and stir in the buckwheat. Cover the pan and simmer gently for 6–8 minutes, stirring occasionally, until the buckwheat is just tender. Don't overcook it or it will become mushy.

3. Leave to stand, covered, for 2–3 minutes, then spread out the buckwheat on a large plate and set aside to cool.

4. Steam the green beans and broccoli in a steamer or a colander placed over a pan of simmering water for 4–5 minutes until tender but still a little crisp.

5. Dry-fry the sesame seeds in a frying pan (skillet) over a medium heat for 1–2 minutes, tossing them gently, until golden brown and fragrant. Remove and leave to cool.

6. Drain the sun-blush tomatoes and cut them into small pieces. Mix with the sprouted seeds, chives, buckwheat and warm broccoli and beans in a large bowl. Pour over the vinaigrette dressing and toss gently. Season to taste with salt and pepper.

7. Divide the salad between 4 serving plates and dot with the goat's cheese. Sprinkle with the chilli flakes and toasted sesame seeds and eat while it's still warm.

OR YOU CAN TRY THIS...

- Use baby plum tomatoes instead of sun-blush ones.

- Sunflower, fennel, cumin or pumpkin seeds also work well in this salad.

- Scatter with crumbled feta or creamy blue cheese if you don't like goat's cheese.

- Experiment with different herbs: mint, tarragon, flat-leaf parsley, coriander (cilantro) and basil.

NICOISE PLATTER

This platter of tasty appetizers is inspired by the flavours of Provence, and includes the rich olive paste – or tapenade as it's called in Nice – to spread onto grilled bread.

SERVES 8
PREP: 40 MIN
COOK: 15 MIN

675g/1½lb baby new potatoes

grated zest and juice of 1 lemon

150ml/5fl oz (⅔ cup) garlic-infused olive oil

2 tbsp chopped fresh parsley

225g/8oz French beans

225g/8oz radishes

4 medium eggs

8 large slices rustic-style gluten-free bread (or 16 small slices)

salt and freshly ground black pepper

lemon wedges, to serve

FOR THE TAPENADE

110g/4oz stoned (pitted) black olives

2 anchovy fillets in oil, drained and chopped

2 tbsp chopped fresh parsley

4 tbsp garlic-infused olive oil

1. Put the potatoes in a pan of cold, salted water and set over a medium heat. Cover and bring to the boil, then simmer for about 15 minutes until a knife inserted into them goes in easily. Drain and leave to cool a little, then stir in half the lemon juice and zest, 4 tablespoons of the olive oil and the parsley. Season well with salt and pepper and set aside.

2. While the potatoes cook, make the tapenade. Using a pestle and mortar or a food processor, grind together the olives, anchovies, parsley and a little pepper until fairly smooth. Gradually blend in the oil. Season with salt and pepper to taste and set aside.

3. Bring another large pan of water to the boil, add the French beans, return to the boil and simmer for 3 minutes. Drain and immediately refresh the beans under cold running water; dry well. Toss the beans with the remaining lemon juice and zest and a further 4 tablespoons of olive oil. Season to taste and set aside.

4. Wash the radishes and trim the leaves and root ends; cut in half if large. Toss with the remaining olive oil.

5. Bring a small pan of water to the boil, add the eggs, return to the boil and simmer gently for 7 minutes or longer if a firmer yolk is preferred. Drain and immediately plunge into iced water to cool. Peel and carefully cut in half.

6. Preheat the grill and toast the bread on both sides. Arrange all the ingredients on one large platter, with the tapenade in the centre. Serve garnished with lemon wedges, and pass around a pot of sea salt for the radishes.

BANG BANG CHICKEN SALAD

This aromatic salad with a hint of chilli is a delicious way to use up leftover chicken from the Sunday roast. Or just buy some ready-cooked chicken and you'll have a quick meal if you serve it with rice or quinoa.

SERVES 4
PREP: 20 MIN
COOK: 2 MIN

100g/3½oz pak choi (bok choy), sliced

2 carrots, cut into thin strips with a potato peeler

2 courgettes (zucchini), cut into thin strips with a potato peeler

100g/3½oz (generous 1 cup) sprouted seeds, e.g. alfalfa

a handful of coriander (cilantro), chopped

a handful of mint or Thai basil, chopped

400g/14oz (generous 3 cups) shredded cooked chicken breast

2 tbsp sesame seeds

salt and freshly ground black pepper

lime wedges, to serve

FOR THE BANG BANG DRESSING:
100g/3½oz (scant ½ cup) crunchy peanut butter

1 red chilli, deseeded and shredded

½ tsp grated fresh root ginger

1 tbsp soy sauce

1 tbsp rice wine vinegar

1 tbsp sesame oil

1 tsp caster (superfine) sugar

4–5 tbsp onion-free chicken stock

◎ ◎ ◎

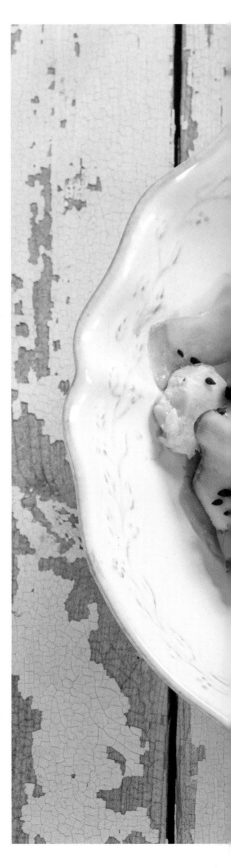

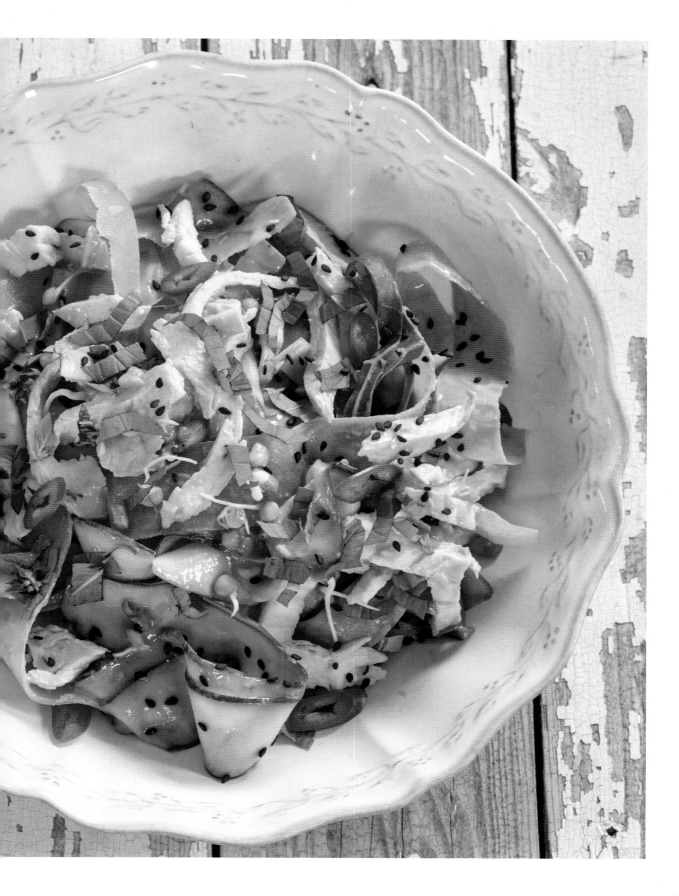

⊙⊙⊙ BANG BANG CHICKEN SALAD

1. Make the bang bang dressing: mix together the peanut butter, chilli and ginger. Stir in the soy sauce, vinegar, sesame oil and sugar. Thin to a pouring consistency with the chicken stock, adding a spoonful at a time.

2. Put the prepared vegetables and sprouted seeds in a large bowl. Add the herbs and chicken, and season to taste.

3. Pour the dressing over the salad and gently toss everything together.

4. Heat a small frying pan (skillet) over a medium to high heat and dry-fry the sesame seeds for 1–2 minutes, tossing them gently, until they release their aroma. Remove before they burn.

5. Divide the salad between 4 serving plates and scatter with the toasted sesame seeds. Serve with lime wedges.

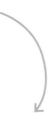

OR YOU CAN TRY THIS...

- ⊙ Use hot Szechuan peppercorns instead of regular ones for extra heat.

- ⊙ Serve the salad with a drizzle of sweet chilli sauce.

- ⊙ For more crunch, mix in some raw red pepper, sugar snap peas or shredded mangetout (snow peas).

- ⊙ Use thin cucumber strips instead of the courgettes (zucchini).

CAVOLO NERO & QUINOA WITH FETA

Cavolo nero is a dark green variety of kale from Tuscany, so dark that the leaves are almost black and hence its name (*nero* is the Italian word for 'black').

SERVES 4
PREP: 10 MIN
COOK: 25 MIN

150g/5oz (scant 1 cup) quinoa (dry weight)

400ml/14fl oz (1¾ cups) onion-free vegetable stock

250g/9oz cavolo nero, stems discarded and leaves shredded

juice of 1 lemon

4 tbsp fruity olive oil

4 tbsp sultanas (golden raisins)

3 tbsp pine nuts

1 small preserved lemon, pulp discarded and rind cut into shreds

a pinch of dried chilli (hot pepper) flakes

100g/3½oz (scant ¾ cup) diced feta cheese

2 tbsp snipped chives

salt and freshly ground black pepper

1. Rinse the quinoa under running cold water. Bring the stock to the boil in a large saucepan and add the quinoa. Reduce the heat to low, cover the pan and simmer for 12–15 minutes until just tender. Turn off the heat and leave to steam in the pan for 5 minutes. Drain and fluff up the quinoa with a fork.

2. Put the cavolo nero, 2 tablespoons water and a good pinch of salt in a saucepan. Cover with a lid and place over a medium to high heat for about 3–4 minutes, shaking the pan occasionally, until the leaves wilt and are slightly tender and the liquid evaporates.

3. Stir the lemon juice, olive oil, sultanas, pine nuts, shredded preserved lemon rind and chilli flakes into the warm quinoa. Gently fold in the cavolo nero, season with salt and pepper and transfer to a serving bowl.

4. Sprinkle with the feta cheese and chives and serve warm.

OR YOU CAN TRY THIS...

- Use spinach instead of cavolo nero – it will turn bright green and wilt in 2 minutes in the pan. Drain well before adding to the quinoa.

- To make the salad more substantial, mix in some roasted vegetables.

- If you can't get cavolo nero, use curly kale instead.

REALLY GREEN QUINOA TABBOULEH

Of course, this isn't a real tabbouleh but it's prepared and flavoured in a similar way. Really refreshing and nutritious, it's delicious served with some griddled or roast chicken.

SERVES 4
PREP: 20 MIN
COOK: 15 MIN

150g/5oz (scant 1 cup) quinoa (dry weight)

400ml/14fl oz (1¾ cups) onion-free vegetable stock

60g/2oz (scant ½ cup) hazelnuts, roughly chopped

2 tbsp pine nuts

100g/3½oz curly kale, roughly chopped

100g/3½oz baby spinach leaves, shredded

60g/2oz wild rocket (arugula), roughly chopped

¼ cucumber, diced

1 small bunch of basil, chopped

FOR THE CHILLI SESAME DRESSING:
1 green bird's eye chilli, finely chopped

2 tsp white sesame seeds

¼ tsp sea salt crystals

4 tbsp fruity olive oil

juice of 1 lemon

1. Rinse the quinoa under running cold water. Bring the stock to the boil in a large saucepan and add the quinoa. Reduce the heat to low, cover the pan and simmer for 12–15 minutes until just tender. Turn off the heat and leave to steam in the pan for 5 minutes. Drain and fluff up the quinoa with a fork. Set aside to cool.

2. Heat a non-stick frying pan (skillet) over a medium heat. Add the hazelnuts and pine nuts and dry-fry, tossing a few times, for 1–2 minutes until fragrant and golden. Make sure they don't burn. Remove from the heat and set aside to cool.

3. Make the dressing: in a pestle and mortar crush the chilli, sesame seeds and sea salt crystals. Gradually add the oil and then stir in the lemon juice until well combined.

4. Put the kale, spinach, rocket, cucumber and basil in a large bowl. Mix well. Add the pine nuts, hazelnuts and quinoa.

5. Pour over the dressing and toss lightly together. Divide the tabbouleh between 4 serving plates.

OR YOU CAN TRY THIS…

- Experiment with different vegetables, including peppery watercress, a few chopped broccoli florets or some courgettes (zucchini) cut into matchsticks.

- Use fresh coriander (cilantro) or mint instead of basil.

- Add some grated lemon zest, lime juice or citrusy sumac to the dressing.

- Stir some capers or sun-blush tomatoes into the salad.

- Crumble some salty feta cheese over the top.

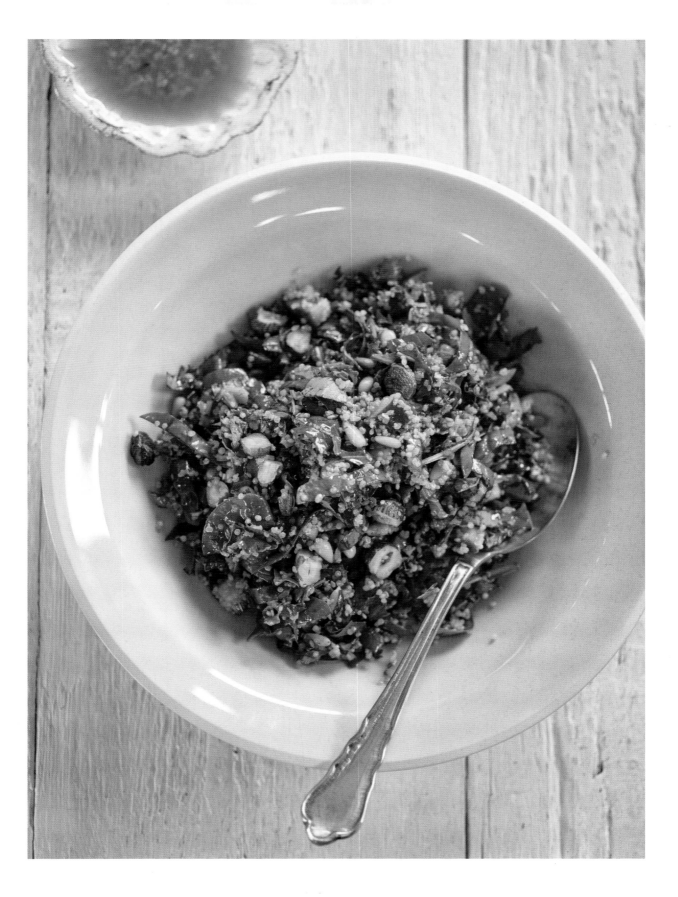

ROAST CHICKEN & RICE SALAD

This recipe uses cold roast or leftover chicken, but you could roast a small chicken and, when cool enough to handle, cut it into pieces and add warm to the salad. Using brown rice gives a nutty flavour and crunchy texture.

SERVES 4
PREP: 15 MIN
COOK: 30–40 MIN

225g/8oz (1 cup) brown rice (dry weight)

200g/7oz sprouted seeds, e.g. alfalfa

1 ripe mango, peeled, stoned (pitted) and diced

500g/1lb 2oz cold roast chicken, cut into strips

a handful of mint, coarsely chopped

a handful of coriander (cilantro), coarsely chopped

salt and freshly ground black pepper

FOR THE THAI DRESSING:
1 red Thai bird's eye chilli, deseeded and shredded

2 tbsp olive oil

1 tbsp sesame oil

2 tbsp nam pla (Thai fish sauce)

juice of 1 lime

1. Put the rice in a saucepan with twice its volume of water and a good pinch of salt. Bring to the boil, then reduce the heat to simmer and cover the pan. Cook gently for about 30–40 minutes until the rice is tender and the liquid evaporates. Check it from time to time to make sure it doesn't stick to the pan, adding more water if necessary.

2. Remove from the heat and set aside, still covered, for 10 minutes before fluffing up the rice with a fork. Set aside to cool.

3. Meanwhile, make the dressing: whisk all the ingredients together in a small bowl or shake in a screwtop jar.

4. Transfer the rice to a large bowl and add the sprouted seeds, mango and chicken. Mix well and then stir in the dressing and chopped herbs.

5. Season with salt and pepper and divide between 4 serving plates.

OR YOU CAN TRY THIS...

- Use white basmati rice instead of brown.

- Mix the chicken, sprouted seeds and mango into cooked quinoa, then toss in the dressing.

- Add some coarsely chopped roasted peanuts to the salad for extra crunch.

- Leftover turkey works equally well or try this with juicy cooked prawns (shrimp).

GRIDDLED AUBERGINE SALAD

This salad is a great accompaniment to grilled (broiled) lamb, chicken, white fish or tofu. Aubergine (eggplant) usually needs a lot of salt, but go easy on it and taste the finished salad first as the feta is quite salty.

SERVES 4
PREP: 5 MIN, PLUS SOAKING
COOK: 20 MIN

2 large aubergines (eggplants)

4 tbsp olive oil

juice of 1 lemon

a pinch of crushed chilli (hot pepper) flakes

225g/8oz ripe baby plum tomatoes

180g/6oz feta cheese, crumbled

a few sprigs of dill, chopped

a few sprigs of flat-leaf parsley, chopped

balsamic vinegar, for drizzling

salt and freshly ground black pepper

1. Cut the aubergines lengthways into slices and place in a shallow bowl. Pour over the olive oil and set aside for 10 minutes to soak.

2. Heat a ridged cast iron griddle pan over a medium heat and cook the aubergine in batches, a few slices at a time, for about 3 minutes each side until tender, golden and striped with the griddle marks. Transfer to a large serving platter.

3. Add the lemon juice, crushed chilli flakes and tomatoes to the pan and heat gently for 2–3 minutes, pressing down on the tomatoes to crush them and release some of their juice. Season with black pepper, and add to the aubergine slices on the serving platter.

4. Scatter the feta over the top and sprinkle with the dill and parsley. Drizzle with balsamic vinegar and serve warm.

OR YOU CAN TRY THIS...

- Top the aubergine salad with pieces of mozzarella or torn burrata instead of feta.

- Add some roasted (bell) peppers or courgettes (zucchini).

- Use fresh basil leaves or coarsely chopped coriander (cilantro).

WARM ROASTED ROOTS SALAD
WITH CRISPY PROSCIUTTO

Root vegetables are naturally sweet and roast well. This simple dish makes a great winter salad and goes well with a gluten-free pasta bake or a simple roasted chicken. Or serve it with a poached or fried egg on top.

SERVES 4
PREP: 15 MIN
COOK: 25 MIN

3 large carrots, peeled

2 parsnips, peeled

3 tbsp olive oil

1 tsp crushed coriander seeds

250g/9oz kale, stalks removed and coarsely shredded

grated zest of 1 small lemon

110g/4oz (1 cup) diced Fontina cheese or mozzarella

8 wafer-thin slices prosciutto or Parma ham

1 tbsp balsamic vinegar

snipped chives, for sprinkling

salt and freshly ground black pepper

1. Preheat the oven to 190°C, 375°F, gas mark 5.

2. Cut the carrots and parsnips into chunky matchsticks. Spread them out in a large roasting tin (pan) and sprinkle over the oil and coriander seeds. Season lightly with salt and pepper.

3. Roast in the preheated oven for 10–12 minutes. Add the kale and lemon zest and stir well to mix the vegetables in the seedy oil. Return to the oven for 10 minutes until the carrots and parsnips are tender and the kale is crisp. Dot with the cheese and pop back into the oven for 2–3 minutes until the cheese is melted.

4. Meanwhile, heat a large frying pan (skillet) over a medium heat. When it's really hot, add the prosciutto and cook for 1–2 minutes until crisp and golden brown. Remove immediately and drain on kitchen paper (towels).

5. Arrange the cheesy roasted vegetables on 4 serving plates, top with the crisp ham and drizzle with the balsamic vinegar. Sprinkle with the chives and serve warm.

OR YOU CAN TRY THIS…

- Use cumin instead of coriander seeds.
- Add a diced red chilli or a pinch of dried chilli (hot pepper) flakes with the kale.
- If you like blue cheese, use gorgonzola instead of Fontina or mozzarella.
- For a more substantial salad, add a small sliced avocado.
- Use naturally sweet swede (rutabaga) instead of parsnips.

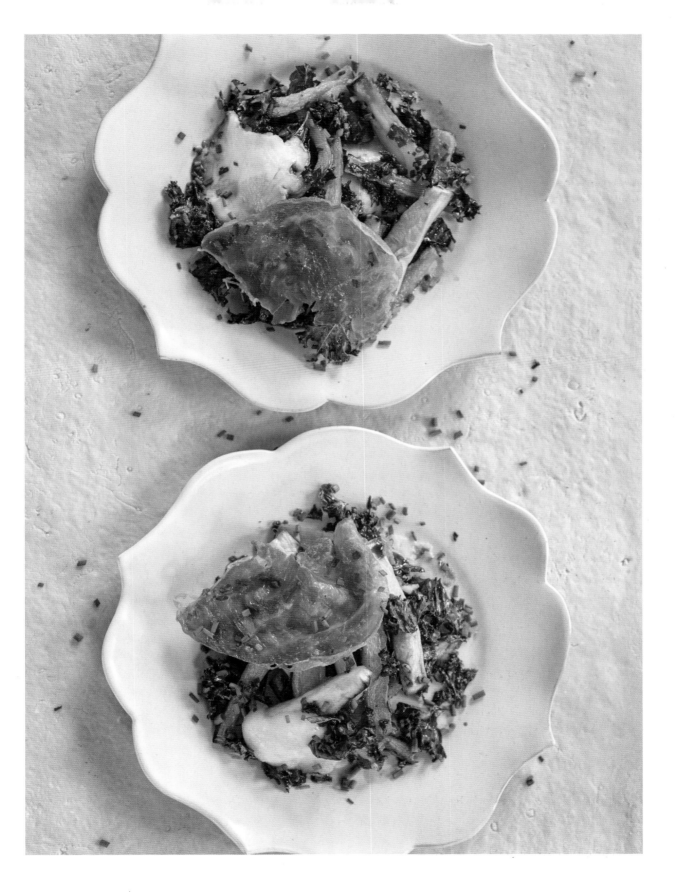

CRUNCHY SEEDY NUTTY FODMAP COLESLAW

You can eat cabbage in moderation on the low FODMAP diet — up to 1 cup of shredded red or white cabbage, which is more than enough to make this spiced healthy coleslaw. To make the chopping, shredding and grating easier, use a food processor.

SERVES 4–6
PREP: 15 MIN
COOK: 5–8 MIN

60g/2oz (scant ½ cup) pecans or walnuts

¼ small red or white cabbage, cored and shredded

1 small head Chinese leaves (Chinese cabbage), shredded

1 small fennel bulb, trimmed and thinly sliced

2 carrots, coarsely grated

4 slices fresh pineapple or 1 ruby red grapefruit, peeled and segmented

a small bunch of chives, snipped

a handful of coriander (cilantro), chopped

juice of 1 orange

FOR THE SEEDY YOGHURT DRESSING:

1 red chilli, deseeded and diced

2.5cm/1in piece fresh root ginger, peeled and diced

2 tbsp olive oil

1 tsp cumin seeds

1 tsp black mustard seeds

150g/5oz (generous ½ cup) 0% fat Greek yoghurt or lactose-free yoghurt

salt and freshly ground black pepper

○ ○ ○

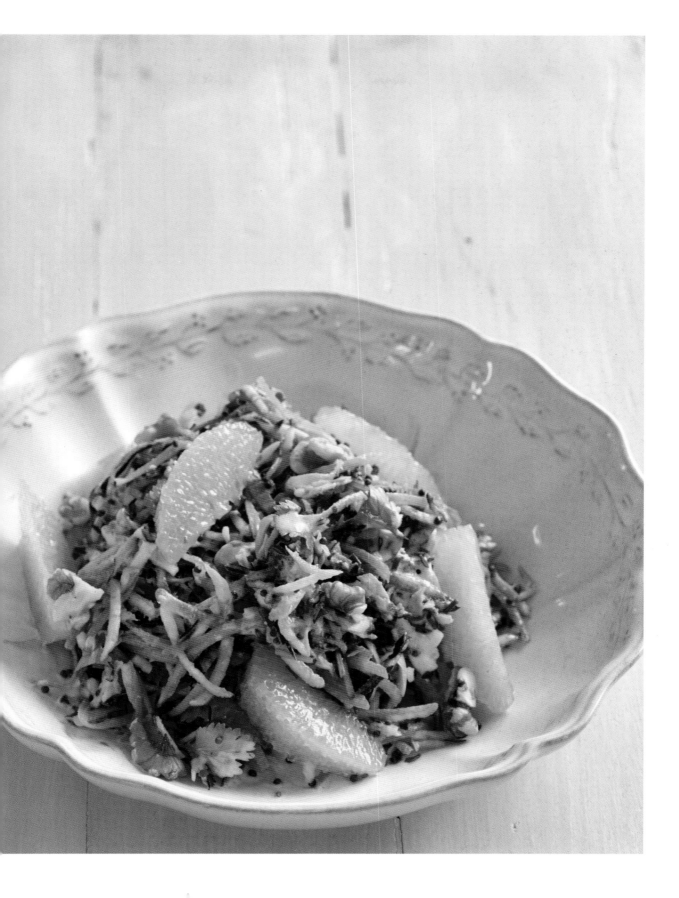

CRUNCHY SEEDY NUTTY FODMAP COLESLAW

1. Set a small frying pan (skillet) over a medium heat and dry-fry the nuts for 1–2 minutes, tossing gently, until golden brown. Remove from the pan and set aside to cool.

2. Put the cabbage, Chinese leaves, fennel, carrots, pineapple or grapefruit and herbs in a large serving bowl. Sprinkle with the orange juice.

3. Make the dressing: gently cook the chilli and ginger for 2–3 minutes in the oil over a low heat. Add the seeds and cook for 1–2 minutes until they release their fragrance. Remove from the heat and stir in the yoghurt. Season to taste with salt and pepper.

4. Gently toss the salad in the dressing until everything is lightly coated. Sprinkle with the toasted nuts and serve.

OR YOU CAN TRY THIS...

- Use hazelnuts instead of pecans or walnuts.

- Orange, clementine or tangerine segments work equally well in this salad.

- Leave out the chilli or use a pinch of dried chilli (hot pepper) flakes instead.

- Toss the salad in a vinaigrette dressing or some plain mayonnaise.

CURRIED ROOT VEGETABLE SOUP

This is a really thick warming soup for a cold winter's day. Serve it with gluten-free bread or crackers. It freezes well, so make double the quantity and cool before sealing in an airtight container and freezing.

SERVES 6
PREP: 20 MIN
COOK: 35 MIN

2 tbsp olive oil

2.5cm/1in piece fresh root ginger, peeled and diced

1 tsp crushed cumin seeds

1 tsp crushed coriander seeds

2 tsp curry powder

2 celery stalks, diced

900g/2lb mixed swede (rutabaga), parsnips, carrots, celeriac (celery root), peeled and diced

1.2 litres/40fl oz (5 cups) hot onion-free vegetable stock

300ml/10½fl oz (1¼ cups) semi-skimmed milk, almond milk or lactose-free milk

2 tsp ground turmeric

1 tsp ground cumin

salt and freshly ground black pepper

natural or lactose-free yoghurt, to serve

2 tbsp chopped coriander (cilantro), to serve

1. Heat the olive oil in a large heavy-bottomed saucepan over a low to medium heat. Add the ginger, crushed seeds and curry powder, stir well and cook for 1 minute.

2. Stir in the celery and diced root vegetables and cook, stirring occasionally, for 10 minutes. Pour in the hot stock and stir well. Bring to the boil, then reduce the heat to a simmer and cover the pan. Cook for 15–20 minutes until the vegetables are really tender.

3. Blitz the soup in batches in a blender or food processor until smooth. Return to the pan.

4. Stir in the milk and ground spices, and season to taste with salt and pepper. Reheat gently over a low heat.

5. Serve in shallow bowls with a swirl of yoghurt, sprinkled with coriander.

OR YOU CAN TRY THIS...

- Add some diced potato with the other root vegetables.

- Substitute a little sweet potato (no more than 300g/10½oz) for one of the root vegetables.

- Use garlic-infused olive oil.

- Sprinkle with snipped chives instead of coriander.

TUSCAN VEGETABLE SOUP

What makes this soup so great is its versatility – you can add almost any FODMAP-friendly seasonal vegetables. Courgettes (zucchini), fennel, chard, green beans and spinach all add to the flavour and nutritional goodness.

SERVES 4
PREP: 15 MIN
COOK: 1 HOUR 10 MIN

3 tbsp olive oil

1 leek, green tops only, chopped

2 celery stalks, chopped

2 carrots, diced

900ml/30fl oz (3¾ cups) onion-free vegetable stock

1 x 400g/14oz can chopped tomatoes

2 large potatoes, cubed

1 tbsp chopped oregano or marjoram

chopped leaves from 1 sprig of rosemary

110g/4oz (1 cup) small macaroni or soup pasta (dry weight)

180g/6oz curly kale, centre ribs and stems removed, leaves shredded

salt and freshly ground black pepper

FOR THE CHEDDAR CRISPS:
110g/4oz (1 cup) grated Cheddar cheese

1. Heat the oil in a large saucepan and cook the leek, celery and carrots over a low heat, stirring occasionally, for about 10 minutes until softened but not coloured.

2. Add the stock, tomatoes and potatoes and bring to the boil. Reduce the heat and add the herbs. Simmer gently for 35–40 minutes. Add the pasta and cook for a further 10 minutes until cooked and all the vegetables are tender.

3. Add the kale and cook for 5 minutes – just long enough to soften a little but not lose its lovely bright green colour. Season to taste with salt and pepper.

4. Meanwhile, make the Cheddar crisps. Preheat the oven to 180°C, 350°F, gas mark 4 and line a baking tray (cookie sheet) with baking parchment. Add 4 circles of grated Cheddar, spaced well apart, and bake for 5 minutes until it melts and spreads – don't let it get too brown. Leave to cool and harden.

5. Serve the soup in shallow bowls topped with the Cheddar crisps.

OR YOU CAN TRY THIS...

- Stir in 1 tablespoon of green pesto just before serving.

- Sprinkle the grated Cheddar over the soup instead of making crisps.

CHICKEN MEAL-IN-A-BOWL SOUP

This warming soup is really substantial and a great way of using up leftover roast chicken and vegetables, so nothing gets wasted. And it's so quick and easy to make after a day at work.

SERVES 4
PREP: 15 MIN
COOK: 20 MIN

2 tbsp olive oil

400g/14oz leftover boiled potatoes, cubed

200g/7oz leftover roast parsnips, cubed

400g/14oz leftover cooked carrots, sliced or cubed

100g/3½oz leftover cooked cabbage or spring greens

leaves from a few sprigs of thyme

900ml/30fl oz (3¾ cups) hot onion-free chicken stock

400g/14oz leftover skinned roast chicken, chopped or shredded

juice of 1 lemon

a handful of parsley, finely chopped

salt and freshly ground black pepper

60g/2oz (½ cup) grated Cheddar or Parmesan cheese, to serve

CHICKEN MEAL=IN=A=BOWL SOUP

1. Heat the oil in a large saucepan over a low to medium heat , add the potatoes, parsnips and carrots and cook gently, stirring occasionally, for 5 minutes.

2. Stir in the cabbage or greens and the thyme. Cook for 1 minute, then add the chicken stock and bring to the boil.

3. Reduce the heat to a simmer and add the chicken, then cover the pan and cook gently for 10 minutes. Stir in the lemon juice.

4. Remove about one-third of the vegetables and chicken with a slotted spoon and set aside while you blitz the soup with a stick blender or in a food processor until smooth.

5. Return the reserved vegetables and chicken to the pan with the puréed soup and heat through gently. Stir in the parsley and season to taste with salt and pepper.

6. Ladle into 4 bowls and sprinkle the grated cheese over the top.

OR YOU CAN TRY THIS...

- Add leftover cooked swede (rutabaga) or even small amounts of broccoli or cauliflower if you can tolerate them.

- Add some chopped tomatoes to the soup.

- Serve the soup with a small swirl of pesto (no more than 1 teaspoon per bowl) or lactose-free yoghurt.

SCALLOP, FRESH PEA & BACON SALAD

Tiny queen scallops are briefly cooked, and mixed with peas, crispy bacon pieces and young spinach leaves. The salad is then drizzled with a creamy mustard dressing. If you buy scallops in their shells, scrub and retain some of the shells to use as a garnish.

SERVES 4
PREP: 10–20 MIN
COOK: 10–12 MIN

180g/6oz smoked lardons (bacon pieces)

450g/1lb shelled queen scallops

150g/5oz shelled fresh peas

225g/8oz young spinach leaves

FOR THE MUSTARD DRESSING

90ml/3fl oz (6 tbsp) light olive oil

1 tbsp lemon juice

1 tsp wholegrain mustard

1–2 tbsp chopped fresh dill or parsley

salt and freshly ground black pepper

1. First make the dressing. Put the oil, lemon juice, mustard and dill or parsley in a screw-topped jar and shake vigorously to combine. Season with salt and pepper to taste.

2. Put the lardons or bacon pieces in a heavy-based frying pan over a moderate heat and fry them in their own fat until crispy. Remove with a slotted spoon and drain on kitchen paper. Set the frying pan over a high heat, add the scallops and sauté for 1–2 minutes. Remove from the pan and allow to cool.

3. Cook the peas in boiling salted water for 5–6 minutes. Drain and refresh under cold running water.

4. Wash and dry the spinach thoroughly, if necessary. Place in a salad bowl with the bacon, scallops and peas and toss to mix the ingredients together. Just before serving, drizzle the dressing over the salad and toss lightly.

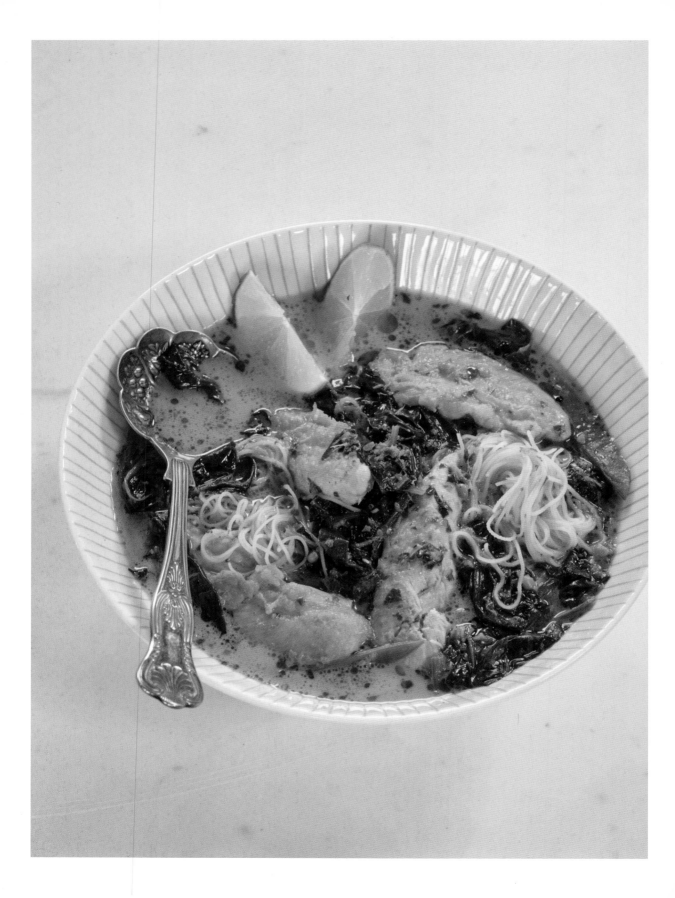

AROMATIC CHICKEN NOODLE SOUP

This spicy soup is always popular, especially on a cold day. All the ingredients are now available from most supermarkets as well as specialist Thai stores and delis.

SERVES 4
PREP: 10 MIN, PLUS SOAKING
COOK: 15–20 MIN

2 green chillies

2 lemongrass stalks, peeled and chopped

1 bunch of coriander (cilantro), plus extra to garnish

1 bunch of Thai basil

grated zest and juice of 1 lime

150g/5oz rice noodles (dry weight)

2 tbsp coconut oil

1 tsp grated fresh root ginger

4 skinned, boned chicken breasts, thickly sliced

900ml/30fl oz (3¾ cups) hot onion-free chicken stock

400ml/14fl oz (1¾ cups) coconut milk

2 tbsp nam pla (Thai fish sauce)

2 fresh kaffir lime leaves, finely shredded

100g/3½ oz mangetout (snow peas), trimmed

100g/3½oz baby spinach leaves

lime wedges, to serve

1. Put the chillies, lemongrass, coriander, basil and lime zest in a food processor or blender and blitz into a thick green paste.

2. Put the rice noodles in a shallow heatproof bowl and cover with boiling water. Soak for 10 minutes, stirring occasionally to prevent them sticking together.

3. Heat the oil in a large saucepan and fry the ginger for 1 minute. Add the chicken and cook over a medium heat for 5 minutes, stirring occasionally, until golden brown.

4. Stir in the spicy green paste and cook for 1 minute, then add the hot chicken stock, coconut milk, nam pla, kaffir lime leaves and mangetout. Simmer for 5–10 minutes or until the chicken is thoroughly cooked. Add the spinach and stir in the lime juice. Cook for 1–2 minutes until the spinach wilts.

5. Drain the rice noodles and divide between 4 shallow serving bowls. Ladle the hot soup over the top, distributing the chicken evenly. Sprinkle with coriander leaves and serve with lime wedges.

OR YOU CAN TRY THIS...

- Use fresh rice noodles which don't require soaking.
- Use snipped chives or Thai mint instead of basil.
- Add halved fine green beans, sliced green pepper or pak choi (bok choy).
- Add some shredded leftover chicken to the soup.
- If you don't have coconut oil, use groundnut (peanut) or even olive oil instead.

COCKLE & POTATO CHOWDER

In this delicious recipe, cooked cockles and creamy, floury potatoes are warmed with a hint of saffron, coriander, orange and thyme. Serve this hearty soup as a substantial starter, or tuck into it as a main meal with plenty of gluten-free bread. As a main course this quantity will serve 4.

SERVES 6
PREP: 15 MIN
COOK: 25 MIN

2 tsp coriander seeds

30g/1oz (2 tbsp) butter

2 carrots, peeled and diced

1 celery stalk, sliced

1 strip pared orange zest

½ tsp saffron strands

450g/1lb cooked cockles, thoroughly drained

600ml/1 pint (2½ cups) milk

480ml/16fl oz (2 cups) fish stock or water

a bouquet garni made from 2 bay leaves, 2 thyme sprigs and a small handful of chives, tied together

675g/1½lb floury potatoes

2 tbsp snipped chives

salt and freshly ground black pepper

4 tbsp double (heavy) cream, to serve

thyme sprigs, to serve

1. Crush the coriander seeds with a pestle and mortar.

2. Melt the butter in a large saucepan. Add the carrots and celery and fry gently for 5 minutes. Stir in the coriander seeds, orange zest, saffron, cockles, milk and fish stock, and add the bouquet garni.

3. Peel and cut the potatoes into small dice, then add to the pan. Bring slowly to the boil, then reduce the heat and cover with a lid. Cook gently for 15–20 minutes until the potatoes are tender. Discard the bouquet garni and orange zest.

4. Transfer half of the soup to a blender or food processor and blitz until smooth. Return to the saucepan, stir in the chopped chives and season with salt and pepper to taste.

5. Ladle into warmed soup bowls and swirl each with a little cream. Sprinkle with small sprigs of thyme.

NOTE: Fresh cockles in their shells are generally difficult to get hold of. If you manage to obtain some, prepare as for mussels, first scrubbing, then cooking briefly in a pan with water; discard any that do not open.

OR YOU CAN TRY THIS…
- Use cooked, shelled mussels instead of cockles.
- Replace the cockles with smoked haddock. Remove the skin and any bones from the fish before adding to the pan.

CARROT, GINGER & MISO SOUP

This quick and easy soup has two stomach-friendly ingredients: ginger and miso. They give the sweet and creamy carrot base a slightly spicy, salty kick.

SERVES 4
PREP: 15 MIN
COOK: 20 MIN

2 tbsp garlic-infused olive oil

4 large carrots, peeled and diced

2 celery stalks, diced

4cm/1½in piece fresh root ginger, peeled and chopped

650ml/22½fl oz (3 cups) rice milk

3 tbsp white miso paste

salt and freshly ground black pepper

1. Heat the oil gently in a large saucepan over a medium to high heat and add the carrot and celery. Sweat for 5 minutes, or until the vegetables have softened. Add the ginger and cook for another 2–3 minutes.

2. Add the rice milk and bring to the boil, then lower the heat and simmer for 10–15 minutes, or until the vegetables are cooked through.

3. Use a stick blender to purée the soup until completely smooth and creamy, then stir in the miso paste and season to taste with salt and pepper. Ladle into 4 bowls to serve.

OR YOU CAN TRY THIS...

⊙ Substitute a little of the carrot with sweet potato (no more than 300g/10½oz).

⊙ Sprinkle with toasted sesame seeds to serve.

THAI RED BEEF CURRY SOUP

Thai curry paste varies considerably in flavour and depth of heat from one manufacturer to another, so go easy and only use a tablespoon at a time, tasting after each addition. Take care to check the ingredients on the label – some brands contain a lot of garlic.

SERVES 6
PREP: 10 MIN
COOK: 30 MIN

2 tbsp coconut oil

1 red (bell) pepper, deseeded and thinly sliced

2.5cm/1in piece fresh root ginger, peeled and shredded

2 tbsp Thai red curry paste

400ml/14fl oz (1¾ cups) coconut milk

900ml/30fl oz (3¾ cups) hot onion-free beef stock

1 tsp palm or brown sugar

juice of 1 lime

1 tbsp nam pla (Thai fish sauce)

100g/3½oz fine green beans, trimmed and halved.

225g/8oz (generous 2 cups) beansprouts

450g/1lb lean sirloin steaks (all visible fat removed)

oil, for greasing

a handful of fresh Thai basil, chopped

1 red chilli, deseeded and shredded

1. Heat the coconut oil in a large saucepan set over a low to medium heat, add the red pepper and cook, stirring occasionally, for about 5 minutes until tender.

2. Add the ginger and cook for 2 minutes, then stir in the curry paste and cook for 1 minute.

3. Stir in the coconut milk and the hot stock and then add the sugar, lime juice, and nam pla. Simmer gently over a low heat for 10 minutes, then add the green beans and cook for a further 5 minutes. Add the beansprouts to the soup and cook for 2 minutes.

4. Meanwhile, heat a little oil in a frying pan (skillet) or griddle pan over a medium to high heat. Cook the steaks for 2–3 minutes each side for medium rare (longer if you like them well done). Remove and leave for 10 minutes before cutting into strips.

5. Stir the basil into the hot soup and ladle into 6 shallow bowls. Arrange the steak strips on top and sprinkle with the chilli.

OR YOU CAN TRY THIS...

⊙ Add some rice noodles to the soup – follow the packet instructions.

⊙ Use Thai green curry paste instead of red.

⊙ You can make a green chicken curry version with green curry paste and 450g/1lb skinned chicken breasts.

⊙ Make a seafood version with onion-free fish stock and fish or shellfish, e.g. white fish fillets, prawns (shrimp), queen scallops and baby squid.

STEAK RAMEN
WITH RICE NOODLES

You don't need onions and mushrooms to make a fantastic ramen. This FODMAP-friendly version is packed with flavour and makes a filling meal in a bowl.

SERVES 4
PREP: 15 MIN
COOK: 12 MIN

250g/9oz rice noodles (dry weight)

1 tbsp sesame oil

1 large carrot, cut into thin matchsticks

2.5cm/1in piece fresh root ginger, peeled and shredded

1.2 litres/40fl oz (5 cups) hot onion-free beef stock

2 tbsp miso paste

2 tbsp gluten-free tamari

1 tsp mirin (rice wine)

200g/7oz pak choi (bok choy), trimmed and sliced

100g/3½oz mangetout (snow peas), trimmed

100g/3½oz (1 cup) beansprouts

juice of 1 lime

450g/1lb rump or sirloin steak (all visible fat removed), cut into thin strips

snipped chives and coriander (cilantro) leaves, to serve

1. Cook the rice noodles according to the instructions on the packet, then drain well.

2. Meanwhile, heat the sesame oil in a large saucepan set over a medium heat and cook the carrot for 5 minutes until tender. Stir in the ginger and cook for 1 minute.

3. Add the hot stock and stir in the miso paste, tamari and mirin. Simmer for 2–3 minutes and stir in the pak choi, mangetout and beansprouts. Cook gently for 2 minutes – no longer or the pak choi will lose its fresh green colour. Add the lime juice.

4. Meanwhile, cook the steak in a lightly oiled griddle pan for 3–4 minutes, until browned and cooked to your liking.

5. Divide the cooked noodles between 4 shallow bowls and pour the soup over them. Arrange the steak on top and sprinkle with the chives and coriander.

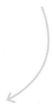

OR YOU CAN TRY THIS…

- Use cubed chicken breasts instead of beef and cook with the carrot and ginger. Add chicken stock instead of beef stock.

- Vegetarians can substitute tofu for the beef.

- You can also add trimmed baby spinach leaves or nori seaweed sheets, cut into strips.

- Sprinkle with a pinch of chilli (hot pepper) flakes just before serving.

SALMON SASHIMI
WITH CUCUMBER
& CARROT SALAD

You'll need the best and freshest salmon you can find – wild salmon is better than farmed. Keep the salmon in the fridge until you're ready to prepare the sashimi. Always wash your hands before and after handling raw fish.

SERVES 4
PREP: 25 MIN, PLUS MARINATING

300g/10½oz salmon fillet (with skin)

120ml/4fl oz (½ cup) light soy sauce, plus extra for drizzling

2 tsp mirin (rice wine)

1 tbsp lime juice

2.5cm/1in piece fresh root ginger, peeled and cut into shreds

85g/3oz baby carrots, cut into thin matchsticks

8 radishes, sliced and cut into matchsticks

¼ cucumber, peeled, deseeded and cut into matchsticks

a handful of coriander (cilantro), chopped

boiled sushi rice, to serve

FOR THE DRESSING:
1 tbsp sunflower oil

2 tbsp lime juice

2 tsp whole-grain mustard

1 tsp caster (superfine) sugar

1. Mix all the dressing ingredients together and blend until smooth.

2. Pick the salmon over carefully, removing any small bones you can find. Place the whole fillet in a rectangular dish or container.

3. Mix together the soy sauce, mirin and lime juice and pour over the salmon. Cover and leave in the fridge for about 45 minutes, turning the salmon frequently in the soy marinade.

4. Remove the salmon from the marinade, pat dry with kitchen paper (towels) and wrap in cling film (plastic wrap). Chill in the refrigerator until you're ready to eat.

5. Just before serving, prepare the salad vegetables (ginger, carrots, radishes and cucumber) and toss them lightly in the dressing with the coriander.

6. Peel off and discard the salmon skin. Using a very sharp knife, cut the salmon into thin slices and arrange them on 4 serving plates. Drizzle with soy sauce and top with the dressed cucumber and carrot salad. Serve with boiled sushi rice.

OR YOU CAN TRY THIS...

- Use mackerel, sea bass or halibut fillets instead of salmon.

- Serve the sashimi with wasabi, daikon radish or pickled ginger.

- Sprinkle with toasted sesame seeds and top with chives.

- Use sesame oil instead of sunflower oil for the dressing.

- Orange or lemon juice can be substituted for lime.

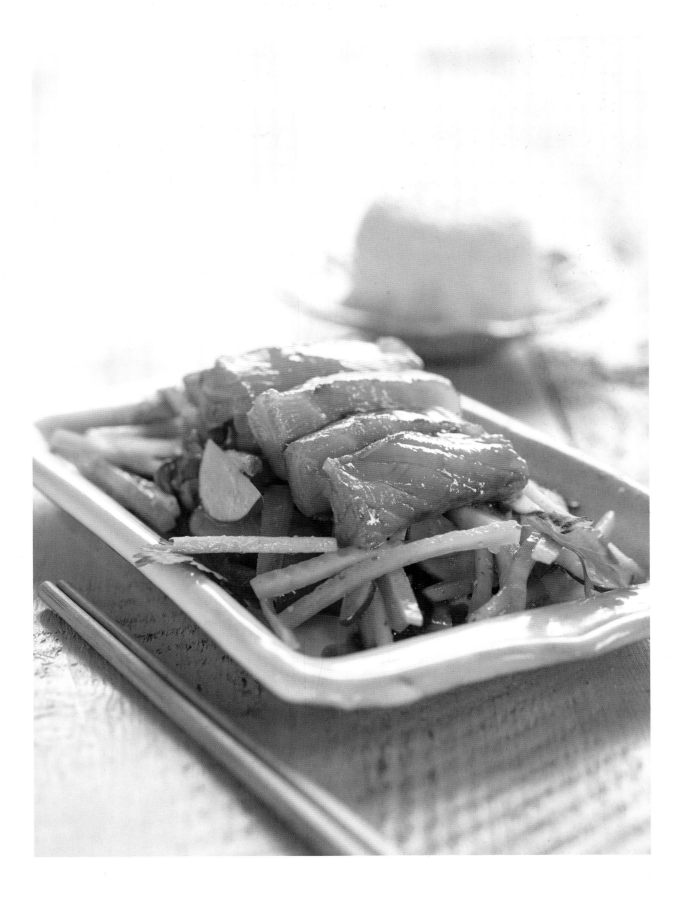

SMOKED SALMON TORTILLA

This makes an economical meal if you use a packet of trimmings rather than the top-quality sliced smoked salmon. You can also eat it warm for breakfast, brunch or supper, or cold as a packed lunch.

SERVES 4
PREP: 10 MIN
COOK: 20–25 MN

1 tbsp olive oil

1 medium carrot, diced

2 celery sticks, diced

100g/3½oz (1 cup) cooked peas

8 free-range medium eggs

1 small bunch of dill, chopped

200g/7oz smoked salmon, cut into thin strips

salt and freshly ground black pepper

1. Heat the oil in a large non-stick frying pan (skillet) over a low to medium heat. Cook the carrot and celery, stirring occasionally, for about 5 minutes until tender. Stir in the peas.

2. Meanwhile, beat the eggs in a clean bowl and stir in the dill, smoked salmon and a little salt and pepper.

3. Pour the egg mixture into the pan and stir into the vegetables. Reduce the heat as low as it can go and cook gently for 10–15 minutes until the tortilla is set and golden underneath and the top is beginning to set, too.

4. Meanwhile, preheat a grill (broiler) until it's really hot. Pop the pan underneath for a few minutes until the top of the tortilla is set and golden brown.

5. Slide it out of the pan onto a plate or board. Leave to cool for 5 minutes, then cut into wedges.

PIPERADE WITH PEPPERS & TOMATOES

Another versatile dish that can be served for brunch, lunch or even supper with a crisp green salad, piperade is a colourful take on scrambled eggs. This traditional speciality comes from the Basque region in southwest France, close to the Spanish border.

SERVES 4
PREP: 10 MIN
COOK: 25 MIN

2 tbsp olive oil

1 red (bell) pepper, deseeded and thinly sliced

1 green (bell) pepper, deseeded and thinly sliced

1 yellow (bell) pepper, deseeded and thinly sliced

500g/1lb 2oz ripe tomatoes, skinned and chopped

a good pinch of sugar

8 medium free-range eggs

2 tbsp chopped flat-leaf parsley, to sprinkle

salt and freshly ground black pepper

gluten-free bread, to serve

1. Heat the olive oil in a large non-stick frying pan (skillet) set over a low heat. Add the peppers and cook gently for about 10 minutes until really tender.

2. Stir in the tomatoes and cook over a medium heat for about 10 minutes until the sauce reduces and the juices evaporate. Add the sugar and season to taste with salt and pepper. Remove about three-quarters of the mixture and keep warm, leaving the remainder in the pan.

3. Beat the eggs in a bowl with some seasoning and pour into the frying pan. Stir with a wooden spoon over a low heat until the eggs start to set. Remove the pan from the heat immediately.

4. Gently stir the egg mixture into the warm peppers and tomatoes, and divide between 4 serving plates. Sprinkle with parsley and eat with crusty bread.

OR YOU CAN TRY THIS…

- Use garlic-infused olive oil.
- Add a diced red chilli or a pinch of dried chilli (hot pepper) flakes.
- Serve topped with a slice of Bayonne ham, as the French do.
- Use roasted or griddled peppers to give the sauce a smoky flavour.
- Add some crisp bacon lardons or pancetta to the sauce.

LOW FODMAP SUSHI

Sushi is really healthy and the good news is that on a low FODMAP regime you can still eat it and even make it yourself – it's surprisingly quick and easy to prepare and tastes delicious. Here are two options: one with prawns (shrimp) and the other with smoked salmon.

SERVES 4–8
PREP: 20 MIN
COOK: 10–15 MIN

300g/10½oz (1¼ cups) sushi rice (dry weight)

2 tbsp rice vinegar

1 tsp sugar

100g/3½oz (¾ cup) peeled cooked prawns (shrimp), roughly chopped OR thinly sliced good-quality smoked salmon

1–2 tsp wasabi, plus extra to serve

4 sheets nori seaweed

1 small ripe avocado

a handful of coriander (cilantro), roughly chopped

light soy sauce, to serve

1. Cook the rice according to the directions on the packet – it will take 10–15 minutes until it's tender and all the water has been absorbed. Stir in the vinegar and sugar, cover the pan and leave to cool until the rice is at room temperature.

2. If using prawns, mix with the wasabi in a bowl – add 1 teaspoon wasabi and taste before adding another as it is extremely hot.

3. Place each nori sheets, shiny-side down, on a bamboo sushi mat or work surface covered with cling film (plastic wrap). Spread the cooled rice over the sheets, leaving a 1cm (½in) border along the long edges.

4. Halve, stone (pit) and peel the avocado and slice it very thinly. Arrange the wasabi prawns on top of the rice, then cover with the coriander and avocado. If using smoked salmon, lay the salmon slices over the rice and then top with the coriander and avocado in the same way; dot a little wasabi on top before rolling.

5. Using the cling film or sushi mat, lift the long bottom edge of one nori sheet over the filling and roll up firmly towards the top, pressing down as you do so. When you reach the top, moisten the edge of the nori with water to seal. Repeat with the remaining sheets to make 4 rolls. If wished, wrap the rolls in cling film in the fridge until ready to serve.

6. Cut each roll into 8 rounds and serve with wasabi and soy sauce for sprinkling or dipping.

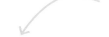

OR YOU CAN TRY THIS...

- Dice the avocado or mash it with the wasabi and a squeeze of lemon juice.

- Add some cucumber, sliced into very thin strips.

- Substitute long fresh chives for the chopped coriander.

SPRING VEGETABLE OMELETTE

You can eat this omelette for lunch, a light supper or brunch. Vary the FODMAP permissible vegetables according to the season and what's available.

SERVES 4
PREP: 15 MIN
COOK: 15–20 MIN

12 baby carrots, trimmed and halved

12 baby turnips

200g/7oz baby leaf spinach

2 tbsp olive oil

6 wafer-thin slices prosciutto or Parma ham

6 large free-range eggs

60g/2oz (½ cup) grated Parmesan cheese

8 baby plum tomatoes

a handful of wild rocket (arugula)

1–2 tsp vinaigrette dressing

salt and freshly ground black pepper

OR YOU CAN TRY THIS…

- Add some chopped parsley, chives, tarragon, basil or dill.

- Use grated Cheddar instead of Parmesan.

- Crumble a crisp-fried streaky bacon rasher (slice) over each serving, instead of prosciutto.

- Add some cooked courgette (zucchini) or even some roasted (bell) peppers.

1. Cook the baby carrots and turnips in a pan of boiling water for 4–5 minutes until just tender. Drain and set aside.

2. Put the spinach in a colander and pour some boiling water over it. Drain and press down with a saucer to squeeze out any excess liquid. Set aside.

3. Heat a little of the oil in a large, deep non-stick frying pan (skillet), set over a medium heat. Add the prosciutto and fry for 1–2 minutes on each side until crisp and golden brown. Remove and drain on kitchen paper (towels).

4. Beat the eggs in a bowl with the Parmesan and a little salt and pepper.

5. Heat the remaining oil in the frying pan and add the cooked carrots and turnips. Scatter the spinach on top and cook over a low heat for 1 minute.

6. Pour in the beaten egg mixture and arrange the tomatoes on top. Cook very gently for about 5 minutes until the omelette sets underneath. Place the pan under a preheated hot grill (broiler) to brown and set the top.

7. Cut the omelette into quarters and transfer to 4 serving plates. Top with the rocket drizzled with vinaigrette and the crispy prosciutto, torn into small pieces.

SPINACH & RICE SOUP
WITH POACHED EGGS

This is a take on a classic Italian soup, where traditionally eggs and spinach are whisked together, then stirred into a hot stock to flavour and thicken it. Serve it topped with a soft poached egg, so that as you put your spoon into the soup the yolk breaks and mingles with the soup – it's delicious!

SERVES 4
PREP: 20 MIN
COOK: 40 MIN

30g/1oz (2 tbsp) butter

4 tbsp garlic-infused olive oil

1 tsp ground coriander

110g/4oz Arborio rice (dry weight)

150ml/5fl oz (⅔ cup) dry white wine

1.2 litres/40fl oz (5 cups) onion-free chicken or vegetable stock

4 small eggs

350g/12oz spinach leaves

4 tbsp chopped fresh parsley

2 tbsp snipped chives

salt and freshly ground black pepper

cayenne pepper, to serve

freshly grated Parmesan cheese, to serve

1. Melt the butter in a saucepan with the oil and ground coriander. Add the rice and stir-fry for 1–2 minutes until all the grains are glossy. Pour in the wine and boil rapidly for 3 minutes.

2. Add the stock, bring to the boil, cover and simmer over a low heat for 20 minutes until the rice is almost tender.

3. Heat 5–7.5cm/2–3in depth of water in a small saucepan until it reaches simmering point. Very carefully break the eggs into the water to sit closely together. Return the water to a gentle simmer and cook until the egg whites are just set. Turn off the heat and cover the pan with a lid.

4. Roughly shred the spinach leaves and stir into the soup with the parsley and chives. Cook for 2–3 minutes until the spinach has wilted and season with salt and pepper to taste.

5. Spoon the soup into warmed bowls and carefully top each serving with a poached egg. Sprinkle with a little cayenne and plenty of freshly grated Parmesan. Serve at once.

OR YOU CAN TRY THIS...

⊙ Substitute the spinach with escarole (a bitter salad leaf).

⊙ Omit the poached eggs and serve the soup topped with a little pesto (no more than a teaspoon per person).

DILL PAPPARDELLE
WITH SMOKED SALMON

It's difficult to find fresh pasta that's wheat-free and low-FODMAP, so have this basic recipe on standby. You can roll the pasta dough out by hand, or pop it through a pasta machine, if you have one.

SERVES 4
PREP: 25 MIN
COOK: 3 MIN

180g/6oz (scant 1½ cups) white rice flour, plus extra
   for dusting

50g/1¾oz (scant ½ cup) tapioca flour

1 tbsp xanthan gum

3 large eggs

1 tsbp olive oil

¼ tsp salt

fronds from a small bunch of dill, roughly chopped,
   plus extra sprigs to serve

60g/2oz (4 tbsp) butter

finely grated zest of ½ lemon

200g/7oz smoked salmon, cut into thin strips

salt and freshly ground black pepper

fresh green salad and lemon wedges, to serve

○ ○ ○

DILL PAPPARDELLE

1. Combine the flours, xanthan gum, eggs, olive oil and salt in a food processor and blitz until just coming together. Add the dill fronds and blitz again until it all comes together into a ball of dough.

2. Transfer the dough to a floured surface and knead for a few minutes until smooth. Divide the dough into 2 pieces and wrap one with cling film to prevent it drying out. With a flour-dusted rolling pin, roll out the other ball of dough to as thin a sheet as you possibly can – be aware that it will swell on cooking, so it needs to be almost paper thin before you start to cook it. (You could put the dough through a pasta machine if you have one.)

3. Using a sharp knife, cut strips of pasta about 2cm/¾in thick and dust them in a little flour to stop them sticking together. Repeat with the other ball of dough, rolling it out and cutting into thick strips.

4. Get a large pan of salted water boiling. Add the pasta and cook for about 3 minutes until cooked but still a *little al dente*. Drain in a colander.

5. While the pasta is draining, melt the butter in the still hot pasta pan and add the lemon zest. Return the pasta to the pan and toss it in the butter to coat, then add the salmon strips and carefully mix those in too. Season with salt and plenty of black pepper. Divide onto 4 plates and serve sprinkled with more dill fronds, with a green salad and lemon wedges on the side.

OR YOU CAN TRY THIS…

- Use flaked smoked mackerel instead of salmon.

- Mix in some lightly steamed sugar snap peas and long-stem broccoli florets.

BUCKWHEAT-STUFFED MEDITERRANEAN VEGETABLES

You can serve these stuffed vegetables hot, lukewarm or cold – whichever you choose, they're equally delicious. The buckwheat has a pleasant nutty texture and the seeds and pine nuts add crunch. Serve with a salad or griddled chicken or lamb.

SERVES 4
PREP: 15 MIN
COOK: 20 MIN

2 medium aubergines (eggplants)

2 red or yellow (bell) peppers

2 tbsp olive oil, plus extra for drizzling

150g/5oz (1 cup) buckwheat (kasha)

1 courgette (zucchini), diced

3 tomatoes, diced

a small bunch of flat-leaf parsley, finely chopped

30g/1oz (¼ cup) pine nuts

2 tbsp sunflower or pumpkin seeds

grated zest and juice of 1 lemon

60g/2oz (½ cup) grated Cheddar or Parmesan cheese

salt and freshly ground black pepper

1. Preheat the oven to 200°C, 400°F, gas mark 6.

2. Cut the aubergines and peppers in half lengthways through the stalk. Discard the white ribs and seeds inside the peppers. Place them, cut-side up, on a baking tray (cookie sheet) and drizzle with olive oil. Bake in the preheated oven for 20 minutes until tender. Remove and set aside to cool.

o o o

BUCKWHEAT-STUFFED MEDITERRANEAN VEGETABLES

3. Meanwhile, cook the buckwheat according to the instructions on the packet.

4. Heat the 2 tablespoons of olive oil in a frying pan (skillet), add the diced courgette and cook over a low heat for 5 minutes, stirring occasionally, until softened. Turn up the heat and add the tomatoes and parsley. Cook for 4–5 minutes and season to taste with salt and pepper.

5. Dry-fry the pine nuts in a small frying pan (skillet), set over a medium heat for 1–2 minutes, stirring a few times, until golden brown. Remove immediately.

6. Scoop the cooked flesh out of the aubergines and dice it. Stir into the courgette and tomato mixture with the cooked buckwheat, pine nuts, seeds, lemon zest and juice. Check the seasoning.

7. Spoon the buckwheat mixture into the baked aubergine and pepper shells and sprinkle with the grated cheese. Return to the oven for 8–10 minutes until golden brown on top.

OR YOU CAN TRY THIS...

- Add a dash of harissa or hot pepper sauce to the filling.

- For more spice, stir in a spoonful of cumin, fennel or caraway seeds.

TIP
Use the grating blade of a food processor to grate the courgette, instead of dicing.

COURGETTE, SPINACH & FETA FRITTATA

The great thing about frittata is that you can eat it cold the following day. Pack it in a lunchbox and take it to work or college with you, or serve at a picnic. It's the perfect finger food.

SERVES 4
PREP: 10 MIN
COOK: 12–15 MIN

1 tbsp olive oil

2 large courgettes (zucchini), coarsely grated

a handful of mint, chopped

110g/4oz baby spinach leaves

a pinch of dried chilli (hot pepper) flakes (optional)

6 medium free-range eggs

2 tbsp semi-skimmed milk or lactose-free milk

a pinch of smoked paprika

85g/3oz feta cheese, diced

1 tbsp grated Parmesan cheese

salt and freshly ground black pepper

1. Heat the olive oil in a large, deep non-stick frying pan (skillet), set over a low heat. Add the courgettes and cook for 4–5 minutes, stirring occasionally. Stir in the mint, baby spinach and chilli flakes (if using) and cook for 1 minute until the spinach wilts and turns bright green.

2. Beat together the eggs and milk, then season lightly with salt and pepper and the smoked paprika. Stir in the feta.

3. Pour into the pan and cook over a low heat for about 5 minutes until the frittata sets and is golden brown underneath.

4. Sprinkle the Parmesan over the top of the frittata and place the pan under a preheated hot grill (broiler) until golden brown and set on top.

5. Serve hot or, preferably, lukewarm and cut into wedges.

TIP
Use the grating blade of a food processor to grate the courgettes.

OR YOU CAN TRY THIS...

- Use cayenne pepper instead of paprika.

- Add some grated lemon zest.

- Instead of mint, use chives, basil or parsley.

- For a less salty flavour and more creamy texture, use soft goat's cheese instead of feta.

- For a more substantial frittata, cook 2 thinly sliced boiled potatoes with the courgettes before adding the eggs.

QUINOA & SWEET POTATO BURGERS

The mashed sweet potato adds sweetness to these healthy veggie burgers. You can make them in advance and leave them in the fridge to chill for several hours, or even overnight, before cooking them.

SERVES 4
PREP: 45 MIN
COOK: 50 MIN

2 sweet potatoes

110g/4oz (⅔ cup) quinoa (raw weight)

3 tbsp olive oil

1 courgette (zucchini), coarsely grated

110g/4oz (generous 3 cups) chopped spinach

a pinch of dried chilli (hot pepper) flakes, plus extra if needed

45g/1½oz (½ cup) gluten-free dry breadcrumbs

a good squeeze of lemon juice

rice flour or another gluten-free flour, for dusting

salt and freshly ground black pepper

TO SERVE:
4 gluten-free burger buns, split and toasted

salad leaves

sliced tomatoes

sweet chilli sauce, tomato ketchup or chutney (see NOTE below)

NOTE
Go easy on the condiments – no more than 1 tablespoon tomato ketchup, chutney or sweet chilli sauce, provided they don't contain garlic or onion.

1. Preheat the oven to 200°C, 400°F, gas mark 6 and bake the sweet potatoes for about 45 minutes until tender. When they're cool enough to handle, remove their skins and mash the flesh in a large bowl.

2. Meanwhile, cook the quinoa in a pan of pan of lightly salted water. Bring to the boil, then reduce the heat and simmer, covered, for about 20 minutes until tender. Drain well and then return to the pan. Cover with a lid and set aside for 10–15 minutes.

3. Heat 1 tablespoon olive oil in a clean pan and cook the courgette for 1–2 minutes. Mix in the spinach and chilli flakes and cook for 1 more minute, then stir into the sweet potato with the quinoa. Bind the mixture with the breadcrumbs and add the lemon juice. Season to taste with salt and pepper. You should end up with a moist but not too loose mixture – add more breadcrumbs if necessary.

4. Divide the mixture into 4 equal-sized portions and, using your hands, mould them into burgers. Pop them into the fridge for at least 45 minutes to chill and firm up.

5. Just before cooking dust the burgers with flour. Heat the remaining oil in a non-stick frying pan (skillet) over a medium heat and cook the burgers for about 2 minutes on each side until golden brown. Turn them over carefully with a spatula so they don't fall apart.

6. Serve the burgers in toasted burger buns with salad leaves and tomato slices. Top with a small amount of chilli sauce, ketchup or chutney.

OR YOU CAN TRY THIS...

- Use toasted gluten-free muffins instead of burger buns.
- Stir some chopped herbs into the burger mixture – chives, parsley or mint.
- Add some diced feta or buffalo mozzarella.
- Serve with a bowl of lactose-free yoghurt or some fresh tomato salsa.

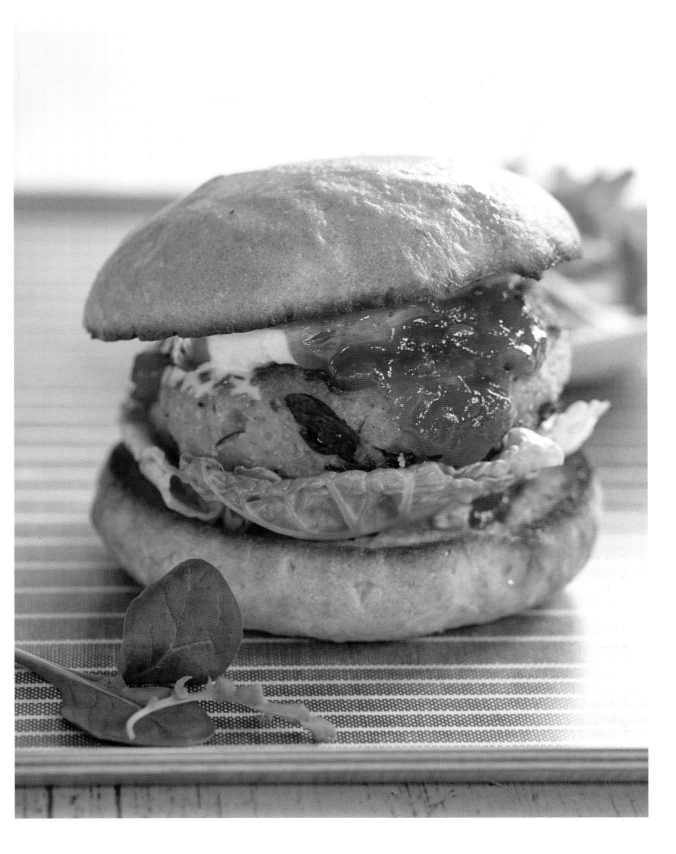

PRAWN, FRESH PEA & PASTA SALAD

This pasta salad is both unusual and incredibly fresh-tasting. When fresh peas are out of season, frozen petit pois make an acceptable alternative.

SERVES 4
PREP: 15 MIN
COOK: 10 MIN

180g/6oz gluten-free pasta, such as penne (dry weight)

110g/4oz shelled fresh peas (about 450g/1lb peas in the pod)

225g/8oz large cooked peeled prawns (shrimp)

2 tbsp chopped fresh mint, plus extra sprigs to serve

1 tbsp chopped fresh chives

60g/2oz hazelnuts, toasted, to serve

FOR THE HAZELNUT DRESSING:

4 tbsp hazelnut oil

2 tbsp vegetable oil

3 tbsp freshly squeezed orange juice

1 tbsp lemon juice

a pinch of sugar

salt and freshly ground black pepper

1. Bring a large pan of lightly salted water to a rolling boil. Add the pasta, return to the boil and cook for 8–10 minutes until barely *al dente* (almost cooked but firm to the bite). Drain well and transfer to a large bowl.

2. Meanwhile prepare the dressing. Place all the ingredients in a screw-topped jar and shake well until evenly combined. As soon as the pasta is cooked, pour over two thirds of the dressing and toss until well coated. Set aside to cool.

3. Blanch the peas in boiling salted water for 1 minute, then drain, refresh under cold water and pat dry. Dry the prawns on kitchen paper and set aside.

4. Assemble the salad just before serving. Add the peas, prawns and herbs to the pasta with the remaining dressing and toss well. Serve at once, topped with the hazelnuts and garnished with mint.

NOTE: Pasta cooking times vary, so always check the packet instructions and remember to undercook by about 1 minute for this recipe, as the pasta will continue to cook as it cools.

OR YOU CAN TRY THIS...
- For an enriched version, add 4 tablespoons mayonnaise to the pasta along with the dressing.

PASTA WITH COURGETTES & BALSAMIC VINEGAR

Courgettes are cooked until meltingly soft and their sweet flavour is enlivened with the addition of balsamic vinegar. Small to medium courgettes work best in this dish and, for the pasta, choose either large ribbons, such as tagliatelle or pappardelle, or shapes (tubes or twists).

SERVES 4–6
PREP: 10 MIN
COOK: 25 MIN

450g/1lb courgettes (zucchini)

3 tbsp pine nuts

4 tbsp garlic-infused olive oil

3 tbsp chopped fresh parsley

400g/14oz gluten-free pasta
(dry weight)

1–2 tbsp balsamic vinegar

6 tbsp freshly grated Parmesan
or pecorino cheese

salt and freshly ground black
pepper

1. Cut the courgettes into thin slices.

2. Heat a large frying pan over a medium to high heat. Add the pine nuts and dry fry, stirring, for 2–3 minutes until lightly browned. Transfer to a small bowl and set aside.

3. Add the oil to the pan. Add the courgettes and increase the heat. Cook, stirring, for about 4 minutes until just beginning to brown.

4. Add the parsley, seasoning and 2 tablespoons water to the pan. Cover, lower the heat and cook gently for 15 minutes, stirring twice.

5. Meanwhile, cook the pasta in a large pan of boiling salted water until *al dente*, or according to packet instructions.

6. Uncover the courgettes and cook for a moment or two over a high heat, stirring gently, until any excess liquid has evaporated. Remove from the heat and sprinkle with the balsamic vinegar and pine nuts.

7. Drain the pasta thoroughly and add to the courgettes with two thirds of the grated cheese. Toss to mix. Serve at once, sprinkled with the remaining grated Parmesan or pecorino.

SUPPERS
=
MEAT

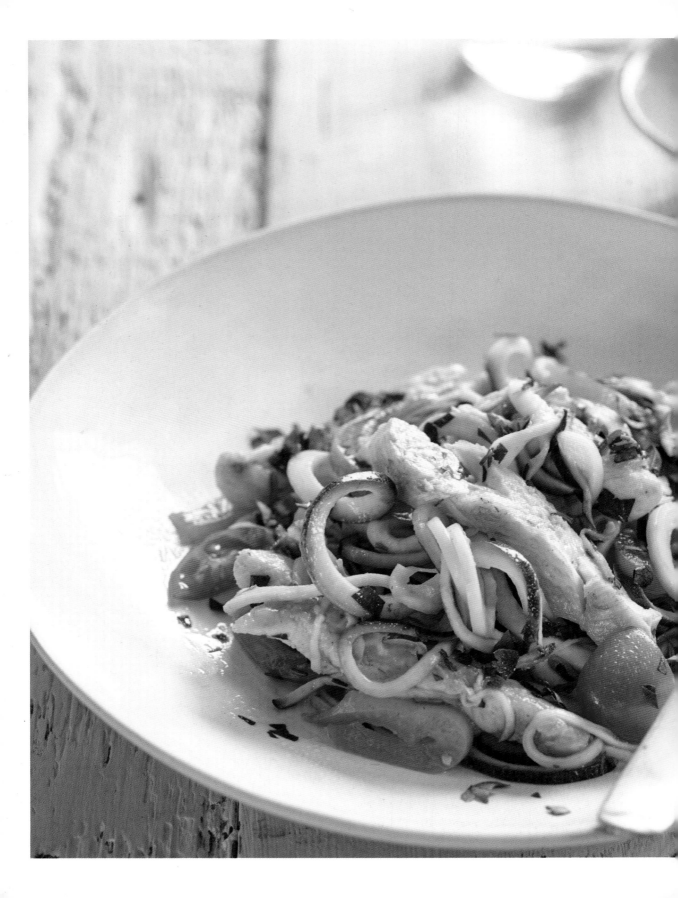

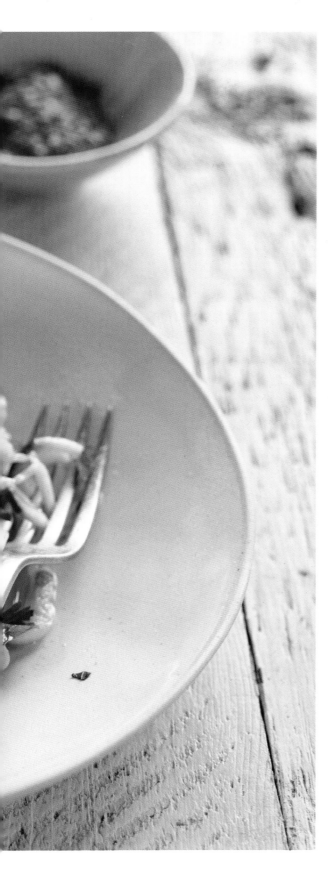

COURGETTI
WITH SEARED
CHICKEN STRIPS

Spiralized vegetables are a healthy and slimming alternative to pasta and have the advantage of being gluten-free. For the best results, use a spiralizer, julienne peeler or mandolin slicer rather than a potato peeler, which will peel long thin lengths from the courgettes (zucchini) but give you much thicker ribbons.

SERVES 4
PREP: 10 MIN
COOK: 30 MIN

4 large courgettes (zucchini), trimmed

2 tbsp olive oil

4 x 110g/4oz skinned, boneless chicken breasts

2 red or yellow (bell) peppers, deseeded and thinly sliced

juice of 2 lemons

210ml/7fl oz (scant 1 cup) onion-free chicken stock

225g/8oz baby plum tomatoes, quartered

a small bunch of parsley, finely chopped

salt and freshly ground black pepper

○ ○ ○

⚬⚬⚬ COURGETTI
WITH SEARED CHICKEN STRIPS

1. Spiralize the courgettes lengthways using blade C, if you have a spiralizer. Alternatively, use a julienne peeler or a mandolin slicer. Set aside.

2. Heat the oil in a frying pan (skillet) and place over a medium heat. Add the chicken breasts to the hot pan and cook for about 15 minutes, turning halfway through, until golden brown and thoroughly cooked all the way through. Remove from the pan.

3. Add the peppers to the pan and cook for about 5 minutes until tender. Add the lemon juice and stock and bring to the boil. Reduce the heat and stir in the tomatoes and half the parsley. Simmer gently for 5–10 minutes until the sauce reduces and thickens.

4. Cut the chicken into thin slices and return to the pan with the courgettes and remaining parsley. Cook for 1–2 minutes until the courgettes are just tender but still retain their shape.

5. Season to taste with salt and pepper and serve immediately.

OR YOU CAN TRY THIS...

- ⊙ Instead of chicken, add grilled (broiled) prawns (shrimp) to the courgetti.

- ⊙ For a more concentrated flavour, add a glug of dry white wine with the stock.

- ⊙ A pinch of dried chilli (hot pepper) flakes makes the dish more spicy.

- ⊙ Chopped coriander (cilantro), chives or basil can be substituted for the parsley.

LEMONY CHICKEN SOUVLAKI

This classic Greek dish is really easy to make and tastes so good. Serve it with green vegetables, such as courgettes (zucchini), kale or green beans, or a Greek salad of tomatoes, cucumber and feta.

SERVES 4
PREP: 15 MIN, PLUS STANDING
COOK: 30 MIN

1 tsp fennel seeds

a good pinch of dried oregano

1 tsp olive oil

grated zest and juice of 1 lemon

500g/1lb 2oz chicken breast fillets, cut into chunks

8 thick woody sprigs of rosemary, most of the leaves removed

2 tbsp chopped parsley

lemon wedges, to serve

FOR THE LEMON ROAST POTATOES:

450g/1lb Charlotte potatoes, halved

2 sprigs of rosemary

a few sprigs of thyme or oregano

olive oil, for drizzling

juice of 1 lemon

salt and freshly ground black pepper

1. Preheat the oven to 200°C, 400°F, gas mark 6.

2. First prepare the lemon roast potatoes: put the potatoes in a roasting tin (pan) and tuck the herbs in around them. Drizzle with plenty of olive oil and pour the lemon juice over them. Season with salt and pepper. Roast in the preheated oven for about 30 minutes until tender and golden brown.

3. Meanwhile, crush the fennel seeds in a pestle and mortar and stir in the oregano, olive oil, and lemon zest and juice. Add the chicken and stir in the lemony mixture until it's coated all over.

4. Thread the chicken onto the sprigs of rosemary (or wooden skewers that have been soaked in water for 30 minutes to prevent them burning). Cover and set aside for 10 minutes.

5. Cook the chicken under a preheated hot grill (broiler) or over hot coals on a barbecue for 10 minutes, turning occasionally, until golden brown and cooked right through.

6. Serve the chicken, sprinkled with chopped parsley, accompanied by the lemon roast potatoes. Squeeze the lemon wedges over the top.

OR YOU CAN TRY THIS...

- Use turkey breast instead of chicken.

- Use largish new potatoes instead of Charlotte potatoes

- Serve with boiled rice instead of potatoes.

- Remove the cooked chicken from the rosemary stems and roll up with some salad leaves, tomatoes and tzatziki in a cornmeal wrap.

SPICY CHICKEN BURGERS

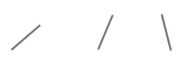

Everyone loves burgers and these healthy spiced chicken ones make a great family supper. If you can't find any minced (ground) chicken in your local supermarket or butcher's, use skinned, boned chicken breasts and blitz in a food processor or blender.

SERVES 2
PREP: 15 MIN, PLUS CHILLING
COOK: 10-12 MIN

500g (1lb 2oz) minced (ground) lean chicken

½ tsp ground cumin

grated zest of 1 lemon

a few sprigs of coriander (cilantro), chopped

a handful of mint, chopped

1 tbsp tomato paste

a dash of harissa paste

olive oil, for cooking

4 gluten-free burger buns or bread rolls

a few rocket (arugula) leaves

1 large beefsteak tomato, sliced

salt and freshly ground black pepper

FOR THE ROCKET (ARUGULA) TZATZIKI:

250g/9oz (1 cup) 0% fat Greek yoghurt

juice of ½ small lemon

4 tbsp chopped fresh coriander (cilantro)

¼ cucumber, diced

30g/1oz wild rocket (arugula), finely chopped

1. Mix the chicken mince, cumin, lemon zest, chopped herbs and tomato paste in a bowl. Add a touch of harissa – it's very hot so don't overdo it. Season with salt and pepper.

2. Divide the mixture into 4 portions and, using your hands, shape each one into a burger. Cover and chill in the fridge for 15–20 minutes to firm them up.

3. Meanwhile, make the rocket tzatziki: mix all the ingredients together in a bowl and season to taste.

4. Lightly brush a ridged grill pan with a little oil and place over a medium heat. Add the burgers to the hot pan and cook for 5–6 minutes on each side until thoroughly cooked inside and golden brown outside.

5. Toast the burger buns lightly and split in half. Add the chicken burgers with a few rocket leaves and sliced tomato. Add a spoonful of the tzatziki and cover with the tops of the buns. Serve immediately.

OR YOU CAN TRY THIS...

- Use Tabasco, hot pepper sauce or even a diced chilli instead of harissa.

- Top the burgers with a slice of cheese and pop under a grill (broiler) to melt.

- Use watercress or spinach to make the tzatziki.

BALSAMIC GLAZED CHICKEN & VEGETABLE TRAYBAKE

This is such a simple supper and by cooking everything in one pan there's hardly any washing up. Serve with a salad or some spinach, kale or steamed green beans.

SERVES 4
PREP: 15 MIN
COOK: 40–50 MIN

2–3 tbsp olive oil oil

4 boned chicken breasts

1 yellow (bell) pepper, deseeded and cut into chunks

1 red (bell) pepper, deseeded and cut into chunks

2 courgettes (zucchini), cut into chunks

300g/10½oz parsnips, peeled and halved or quartered

300g/10½oz baby plum tomatoes

150ml/5fl oz (⅔ cup) onion-free chicken stock

2 tbsp balsamic vinegar

1 tsp fresh thyme leaves

salt and freshly ground black pepper

a handful of parsley, chopped, to sprinkle

balsamic glaze, for drizzling (optional)

1. Preheat the oven to 190°C, 375°F, gas mark 5.

2. Heat the olive oil in a roasting tin (pan) over a medium heat on the hob. Add the chicken and cook for 8–10 minutes, turning occasionally, until browned all over.

3. Remove from the heat and add the peppers, courgettes, parsnips and tomatoes. Pour the stock and balsamic vinegar over the top, sprinkle with thyme and season with salt and pepper.

4. Bake in the preheated oven for 30–40 minutes until the vegetables are cooked and tender.

5. Serve sprinkled with plenty of chopped parsley and a drizzle of balsamic glaze, if you wish.

OR YOU CAN TRY THIS...

- Vary the vegetables – try fennel, aubergine (eggplant), baby carrots and sweet potato (no more than 350g/12oz).

- Sprinkle with fresh rosemary instead of thyme.

- Drizzle with sweet chilli sauce.

CHINESE LEMON CHICKEN

Don't worry that this recipe contains broccoli. Most people on the FODMAP diet can tolerate it in small quantities. Otherwise, use quartered pak choi (bok choy).

SERVES 4
PREP: 10 MIN
COOK: 15 MIN

250g/9oz (1 cup) basmati rice (dry weight)

500g/1lb 2oz skinned chicken breast fillets, cut into strips

1 tbsp sesame oil

2 tsp sesame seeds

2 tbsp sunflower or groundnut (peanut) oil

1 tbsp finely chopped fresh root ginger

150g/5oz long-stem broccoli, trimmed

200g/7oz mangetout (snow peas), trimmed

grated zest and juice of 2 lemons

1 tbsp sweet chilli sauce

2 tbsp light soy sauce

4 tbsp onion-free chicken stock

1 tsp sugar

a small bunch of chives, snipped

1. Cook the rice according to the instructions on the packet.

2. Put the chicken strips in a bowl with the sesame oil. Add the sesame seeds and stir well to coat the chicken.

3. Heat the oil in a wok or deep frying pan (skillet) over a medium to high heat and stir-fry the chicken for 3–4 minutes, until golden brown. Add the ginger and stir-fry for 1 minute.

4. Add the broccoli and mangetout and stir-fry for 1–2 minutes. Stir the lemon zest and juice, sweet chilli sauce, soy sauce, chicken stock and sugar into the wok and cook for 2 minutes or until the liquid reduces and the vegetables are just tender, but still crisp.

5. Divide the cooked rice between 4 shallow serving bowls and spoon the lemon chicken over the top. Sprinkle with chives and serve.

OR YOU CAN TRY THIS...

- For a thicker lemon sauce, mix 1 teaspoon cornflour (cornstarch) with a little water until smooth and stir into the wok at the end, just before serving.

- Serve with rice noodles instead of boiled rice.

THAI ROAST CHICKEN

This dish is quite filling on its own. However you can serve it with steamed or boiled Thai fragrant rice and stir-fried green beans or mangetout (snow peas), if you wish.

SERVES 4
PREP: 15 MIN
COOK: 35–40 MIN

8 boned chicken thighs

1 red (bell) pepper, deseeded and cut into chunks

1 yellow (bell) pepper, deseeded and cut into chunks

1 aubergine (eggplant), cut into chunks

300g/10½oz sweet potato, peeled and cut into wedges

4 tbsp olive oil

freshly ground black pepper

a few sprigs of fresh Thai basil, chopped

FOR THE THAI CURRY PASTE:

1 tbsp Thai green curry paste

2.5cm/1in piece fresh root ginger, peeled and chopped

1 lemongrass stalk, peeled and diced

1 green chilli, deseeded and diced

grated zest and juice of 1 lime

a few sprigs of coriander (cilantro), chopped

1. Preheat the oven to 200°C, 400°F, gas mark 6.

2. Blitz all the curry paste ingredients in a blender until you have a smooth paste. Slash each chicken thigh 2–3 times with a sharp knife and rub the paste into the cuts and all over.

3. Arrange the chicken thighs, peppers, aubergine and sweet potato in a large ovenproof dish or roasting tin (pan). Drizzle with olive oil and grind some black pepper over the top.

4. Bake in the preheated oven for 35–40 minutes, turning the chicken and vegetables once or twice. When the chicken is cooked right through and the skin is crisp and golden, and the vegetables are tender, remove from the oven.

5. Divide the chicken and vegetables between 4 serving plates and serve scattered with chopped basil.

OR YOU CAN TRY THIS...

- Add some courgette (zucchini), baby carrots, parsnip or pumpkin wedges, chunks of swede (rutabaga) or baby plum tomatoes.

- Use red Thai curry paste.

- Sprinkle with chopped coriander (cilantro).

- Serve with a drizzle of sweet chilli sauce.

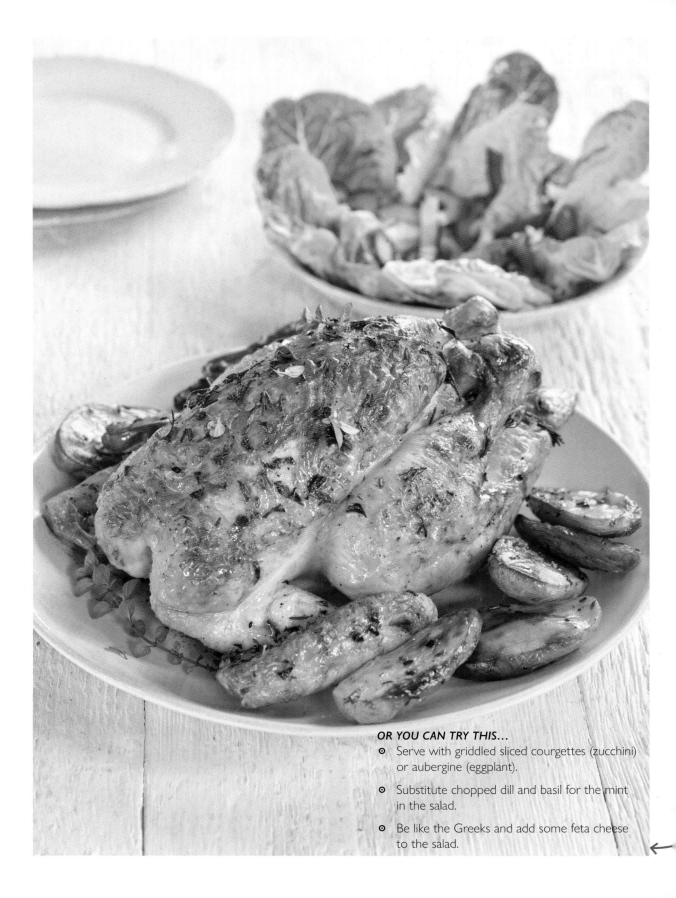

OR YOU CAN TRY THIS...

⊙ Serve with griddled sliced courgettes (zucchini) or aubergine (eggplant).

⊙ Substitute chopped dill and basil for the mint in the salad.

⊙ Be like the Greeks and add some feta cheese to the salad.

GREEK LEMON ROAST CHICKEN & POTATOES

This roast chicken, with its wonderful lemony aroma and flavour, is perfect in spring and summer when you don't want to serve it with stuffing and gravy. And there's minimal washing up, as everything is cooked in the same pan!

SERVES 4
PREP: 10 MIN
COOK: 1 HOUR 20 MIN

1 x 1.35kg/3lb roasting chicken

2 bay leaves

a few sprigs of oregano, thyme or rosemary

675g/1½lb charlotte or new potatoes, halved or quartered

a pinch of crushed chilli (hot pepper) flakes

2 large juicy lemons

4 tbsp olive oil

sea salt and freshly ground black pepper

FOR THE LETTUCE SALAD:

1 cos (romaine) lettuce, separated into leaves

1 green (bell) pepper, deseeded and thinly sliced

1 red (bell) pepper, deseeded and thinly sliced

½ cucumber, thinly sliced

225g/8oz tomatoes, cut into chunks

3 tbsp olive oil

1 tbsp wine vinegar

juice of 1 lemon

a handful of mint leaves, chopped

1. Preheat the oven to 200°C, 400°F, gas mark 6.

2. Wash the chicken under running cold water, then pat dry with kitchen paper (towels) and place in the centre of a large roasting tin (pan). Season with salt and pepper and push the bay leaves and a few of the herb sprigs into the cavity.

3. Arrange the potatoes around the chicken and sprinkle with the chilli. Cut 1 lemon in half and squeeze the juice over the chicken and potatoes. Push the squeezed halves inside the chicken. Cut the other lemon into small wedges and put them in the gaps between the potatoes. Strip the leaves off the remaining herbs and sprinkle over the top. Drizzle the chicken and potatoes with olive oil and carefully pour 4 tablespoons water into a corner of the roasting tin (pan).

4. Roast in the preheated oven for 1 hour 20 minutes, basting the chicken occasionally with the pan juices, and turning the potatoes over as they brown. When the potatoes are cooked, tender and golden brown – even if the chicken is still not cooked – transfer them to a serving dish and keep warm.

5. Check whether the chicken is cooked by inserting a skewer or a thin-bladed knife into the meaty part of one of the thighs. If the juices run clear, it's ready. Remove from the oven, cover with kitchen foil and leave to rest for 10 minutes before carving.

6. Meanwhile, make the salad: mix the lettuce, peppers, cucumber and tomatoes together in a large bowl. Blend the olive oil, vinegar, lemon juice, mint and seasoning and mint by mixing in a small bowl or shaking vigorously in a screwtop jar. Pour over the salad and toss lightly.

7. Carve the chicken and serve with the potatoes, roasted lemon wedges and salad. If you wish, pour some of the warm pan juices over the salad.

CHICKEN SALTIMBOCCA

The name of this Roman dish comes from the Italian for 'jump in the mouth', and it really is delicious. In Italy, thin veal escalopes are traditionally cooked in this way, but chicken works equally well.

SERVES 4
PREP: 10 MIN
COOK: 15 MIN

4 skinned chicken breast fillets
8 fresh sage leaves
4 thin slices Fontina or Swiss cheese
8 wafer-thin slices Parma ham
1 tbsp olive oil
30g/1oz (2 tbsp) unsalted butter
4 tbsp onion-free chicken stock
4 tbsp Marsala
1–2 tbsp crème fraîche or lactose-free cream
salt and freshly ground black pepper
2 tbsp chopped parsley, to serve

FOR THE CRUSHED POTATOES:
500g/1lb 2oz small new potatoes
3 tbsp crème fraîche or lactose-free cream
1 tsp whole-grain mustard
grated zest of 1 lemon

OR YOU CAN TRY THIS...
⊙ Serve with gluten-free pasta or polenta.

⊙ Use dry white vermouth (Noilly Prat) or white wine instead of Marsala.

⊙ Use turkey, pork or veal escalopes instead of chicken.

1. Place each chicken breast between 2 sheets of parchment (waxed) paper or cling film (plastic wrap) and flatten by pounding with a meat mallet or rolling pin until 5mm/¼in thick.

2. Season lightly with black pepper and lay 2 sage leaves on top of each chicken breast. Cover with a slice of cheese and then wrap in 2 slices of Parma ham to enclose the cheese and most of the chicken. Secure if necessary with wooden cocktail sticks (toothpicks).

3. Heat the oil and butter in a large non-stick frying pan (skillet) over a medium heat and cook the chicken for about 5 minutes on each side, until golden brown and cooked through. The chicken is cooked when you pierce it with a sharp knife and the juices run clear. Remove and keep warm.

4. Add the stock and Marsala to the pan and let it bubble away for 4–5 minutes until reduced. Stir in the crème fraîche and season with salt and pepper.

5. Meanwhile, cook the potatoes in a pan of boiling salted water for 12–15 minutes until tender. Drain well and crush coarsely with a fork. Stir in the crème fraîche, mustard and lemon zest, and season to taste with salt and pepper.

6. Serve the chicken in a pool of sauce, sprinkled with chopped parsley and accompanied by the potatoes.

CHICKEN INVOLTINI

Involtini are often served with a tomato sauce, but you can just cook them in oil and butter and add some grated lemon zest and a good glug of white wine or chicken stock to moisten them. Sprinkle with parsley and serve with rice, quinoa or potatoes.

SERVES 4
PREP: 15 MIN
COOK: 25 MIN

4 skinned chicken breast fillets

4 large thin slices Parma ham, all visible fat removed

chopped leaves from 2 sprigs rosemary

4 tbsp grated Parmesan cheese

2 tbsp olive oil

30g/1oz (2 tbsp) butter

4 large ripe tomatoes, roughly chopped

100g/4oz bottled roasted red (bell) peppers, chopped

1 tbsp capers

a pinch of sugar

350g/12oz gluten-free penne or macaroni

salt and freshly ground black pepper

2 tbsp chopped parsley, to sprinkle

1. Place each chicken breast between 2 sheets of parchment (waxed) paper or cling film (plastic wrap) and flatten by pounding with a meat mallet or rolling pin until 5mm/¼in thick.

2. Season lightly with salt and pepper and lay a slice of Parma ham on top of each chicken breast. Sprinkle with the rosemary and Parmesan and roll up tightly like a Swiss roll (jelly roll). Cut each roll in half and secure with a wooden cocktail stick (toothpick).

3. Heat the oil and butter in a large non-stick frying pan (skillet) over a medium heat and cook the involtini for 6–8 minutes, turning often, until golden brown all over. Remove and keep warm.

4. Add the tomatoes, red peppers and capers with a pinch of sugar to the pan and cook for 5 minutes. Place the involtini on top, then cover and cook for 10 minutes until the chicken is cooked through and the sauce has thickened.

5. Meanwhile cook the pasta according to the instructions on the packet and drain well.

6. Remove the involtini and discard the cocktail sticks. Fold the cooked pasta into the tomato sauce and divide between 4 serving plates. Top with the involtini, then sprinkle with parsley to serve.

OR YOU CAN TRY THIS…

- Use turkey or veal escalopes instead of chicken.

- Fill the involtini with chopped basil or parsley and grated Swiss cheese, ricotta or goat's cheese.

- Add some black olives or diced courgettes (zucchini) to the sauce and flavour it with balsamic vinegar.

- Use canned tomatoes instead of fresh.

CHINESE CHICKEN DUMPLINGS
WITH EGG-FRIED RICE

For the best results, the rice should be cooked in advance and chilled — overnight if you like — before stir-frying with the eggs and vegetables. Use only the green tops of the spring onions (scallions) to add an authentic flavour to the egg-fried rice. The dumplings can also be made the day before and left in the fridge until you're ready to cook them.

SERVES 4
PREP: 20 MIN, PLUS CHILLING
COOK: 35 MIN

225g/8oz (1 cup) basmati rice
  (dry weight)

600g/1lb 5oz chicken breast fillets

1 large carrot, coarsely grated

2 tsp grated fresh root ginger,

1 red chilli, deseeded and diced

a handful of coriander (cilantro),
  chopped

2 tbsp soy sauce

2 tbsp sesame oil or groundnut
  (peanut) oil

green tops of 4 spring onions
  (scallions), chopped

2 medium free-range eggs, beaten

110g/4oz (scant ½ cup) canned
  corn kernels

110g/4oz (scant ¾ cup) frozen peas

sweet chilli sauce, to serve

1. Cook the rice according to the instructions on the packet and set aside to cool.

2. Make the chicken dumplings: blitz the chicken, carrot, ginger, chilli, coriander and 1 tablespoon soy sauce in a food processor until minced. Just pulse the mixture about 5 times, so it's chopped rather than a paste.

3. Shape the mixture into small balls, using your hands. You should end up with about 20 dumplings. Chill in the fridge for at least 30 minutes.

4. Cook the dumplings in the top of a steamer for 20 minutes, until cooked through without any pinkness. If you don't have a steamer, arrange them on a heatproof plate in a covered colander or wrapped loosely in foil above a pan of simmering water.

5. Meanwhile, heat the oil in a wok or deep frying pan (skillet) over a medium heat. Add the cold rice and stir-fry for 1–2 minutes until heated through and glistening with oil. Add the eggs, stirring until they scramble and set. Add the corn kernels and peas and stir-fry for 2 minutes. Stir in the remaining soy sauce.

6. Divide the egg-fried rice between 4 serving bowls and place the dumplings on top. Serve with sweet chilli sauce.

OR YOU CAN TRY THIS...

- Instead of coriander, use chopped parsley or chives in the dumplings.

- Leave out the carrot, add 60g/2oz (½ cup) shredded Chinese leaves (Chinese cabbage).

- For a Thai flavour, substitute nam pla (Thai fish sauce) for the soy sauce.

CHICKEN
WITH LIME & GINGER MAYO

If you have enough time, it's well worth making your own mayonnaise for this; in which case, you will probably want to add less lime juice at stage 6.

SERVES 6
PREP: 30 MIN
COOK: 1½ HOURS

7.5cm/3in piece fresh root ginger

1 chicken, about 1.6 kg/3½lb

1 bouquet garni

300ml/10fl ½oz (1¼ cups) dry
    white wine

3 limes, plus extra wedges
    to serve

1 Little Gem lettuce (or cos
    lettuce heart)

8 spring onions (scallions),
    green parts only

300g/10½oz mayonnaise

salt and freshly ground black
    pepper

1 small cantaloupe melon,
    deseeded and sliced,
    to serve

mixed salad leaves and herbs,
    to serve

1. Cut a small piece off the ginger and reserve. Crush the remainder with a rolling pin; there's no need to peel it. Put the chicken into a saucepan in which it fits snugly. Add the crushed ginger, bouquet garni, wine and the pared zest and juice of 1 lime. Pour over enough water just to cover the chicken. Cover with a lid, then bring to the boil and simmer gently for about 1½ hours or until the chicken is tender.

2. Skim off any scum. Leave the chicken to cool in the liquid.

3. Remove the chicken from the pan. Strain the liquid into a wide saucepan and boil rapidly until reduced to about 150ml/5fl oz (⅔ cup).

4. Meanwhile, remove the cooked chicken from the carcass, discarding all skin and bone. Cut the meat into large bite-sized pieces.

5. Trim the lettuce and shred it very finely. Chop the spring onion greens finely. Add both to the reduced liquid and cook for 1 minute, or until the lettuce is just wilted and the onion greens are softened. Transfer to a blender and purée until smooth. Let cool completely.

6. Peel and grate the reserved ginger. Finely grate the zest from the remaining limes. Add the ginger and lime zest to the cooled puréed mixture. Fold in the mayonnaise. Add the juice of 1 lime, or to taste. Season generously with salt and pepper.

7. Pour the lime and ginger mayo dressing over the chicken and toss gently together to coat all the pieces of chicken.

8. Arrange the chicken on a bed of mixed salad leaves and herbs. Scatter with the melon slices and garnish with lime wedges.

CHICKEN NASI GORENG

You can cook the rice specially for this Indonesian dish or use leftover boiled or steamed rice.

SERVES 4
PREP: 15 MIN
COOK: 15 MIN

225g/8oz (1 cup) basmati rice (dry weight)

3 medium free-range eggs

2 tbsp vegetable or groundnut (peanut) oil

1 red (bell) pepper, deseeded and thinly sliced

1 yellow (bell) pepper, deseeded and thinly sliced

1 fresh red chilli, deseeded and diced

1 tsp finely chopped fresh root ginger

400g/14oz chicken breast fillets, sliced

2 tbsp curry paste

110g/4oz pak choi (bok choy), shredded

2 tbsp soy sauce

¼ cucumber, cut into thin matchsticks

salt and freshly ground black pepper

1. Cook the rice according to the instructions on the packet.

2. Beat the eggs and season with salt and pepper. Heat a teaspoon of oil in a wok or non-stick deep frying pan (skillet) over a medium heat. Add half the beaten egg mixture to the hot pan, swirling it around to make an omelette. When set and golden underneath, flip it over and cook the other side. Slide out onto a plate, roll up tightly and cool before slicing thinly, so you end up with omelette ribbons. Repeat with the remaining beaten egg.

3. Heat the remaining oil in the wok or pan and stir-fry the peppers, chilli, ginger and chicken for 3–4 minutes. Stir in the curry paste and pak choi and stir-fry for 2 minutes, before adding the cooked rice and soy sauce. Stir-fry for 2 minutes.

4. Divide between 4 shallow serving bowls and top with the omelette ribbons and cucumber. Serve immediately.

OR YOU CAN TRY THIS...

- Add some small peeled, cooked prawns (shrimp) with the curry paste.

- Fold in some chopped coriander (cilantro) just before serving.

- Instead of omelette ribbons, top each portion of nasi goreng with a fried egg. Serve it for brunch.

- Add some fine green beans and serve with a drizzle of chilli sauce or kicap manis (thick sweet Indonesian soy sauce).

- Flavour with nam pla (Thai fish sauce), not soy.

LEMONY CHICKEN & MOZZARELLA PARCELS

This Italian supper dish is quick and easy to make. It's versatile, too; you can use thin turkey, pork or veal escalopes instead of chicken.

SERVES 4
PREP: 10 MIN
COOK: 15 MIN

4 skinned chicken breast fillets

8 tsp green pesto

300g/10½oz buffalo mozzarella

gluten-free flour, for dusting

2 tbsp olive oil

15g/½oz (1 tbsp) unsalted butter

120ml/4fl oz (½ cup) white wine

120ml/4fl oz (½ cup) onion-free chicken stock

4 tbsp lemon juice

3 tbsp chopped parsley

salt and freshly ground black pepper

potatoes or gluten-free pasta, to serve

rocket (arugula) or watercress, to garnish

1. Put each chicken breast between 2 sheets of parchment (waxed) paper or some cling film (plastic wrap) and beat with a rolling pin or meat mallet until about 5mm/¼in thick. Cut each flattened breast in half.

2. Spread each piece of chicken with a teaspoon of pesto. Cut the mozzarella into 8 slices and place one on each chicken piece. Roll up like a cigar and secure with a wooden cocktail stick (toothpick). Season lightly with salt and pepper and dust with flour.

3. Heat the oil and butter in a large non-stick frying pan (skillet) over a medium heat and sauté the chicken parcels for about 8–10 minutes, turning occasionally, until golden brown all over and thoroughly cooked with no pinkness. Remove and keep warm.

4. Add the wine to the pan and turn up the heat, stirring with a wooden spoon to scrape any brown bits off the bottom. Add the stock and lemon juice and reduce the heat to medium. Cook, stirring occasionally, for about 5 minutes until the liquid reduces. Stir in the parsley and check the seasoning.

5. Arrange 2 chicken parcels on each serving plate and pour the sauce over the top. Serve immediately with potatoes or pasta, garnished with rocket or watercress.

OR YOU CAN TRY THIS...

- Instead of pesto and mozzarella roll the chicken around some sliced Swiss cheese and chopped herbs or sun-dried tomato paste and grated Parmesan.

- Use Marsala rather than white wine for a sweeter sauce.

STEAK TAGLIATA
WITH ROASTED SWEDE 'CHIPS'

For an authentic tagliata the steaks should be really pink and rare inside and well coloured on the outside. Don't waste any leftover pan juices – pour them into the dressing.

SERVES 4
PREP: 15 MIN
COOK: 20 MIN

4 x 225g/8oz lean sirloin steaks

3 tbsp olive oil, plus extra for brushing

1 tbsp balsamic vinegar

juice of 1 lemon

1 tsp Dijon mustard

180g/6oz rocket (arugula)

180g/6oz baby plum tomatoes, halved

60g/2oz Parmesan cheese, shaved with a potato peeler

salt and freshly ground black pepper

FOR THE ROASTED SWEDE (RUTABAGA) CHIPS:

1 large swede (rutabaga)

a few sprigs of rosemary

a few sage leaves, torn

sea salt crystals

olive oil, for drizzling

1. Preheat the oven to 200°C, 400°C, gas mark 6.

2. Make the swede chips: peel the swede and cut into 'chips' ('fries'), which are not too thin or too chunky. Spread them out on a baking tray (cookie sheet) and sprinkle with the herbs and a little sea salt. Drizzle olive oil over them and toss to coat well.

3. Roast in the preheated oven for about 20 minutes, until the chips are golden brown and tender.

4. Meanwhile, brush the steaks with olive oil and season with salt and pepper. Heat a griddle pan or heavy frying pan (skillet) over a high heat until it's really hot. Depending on how you like your steaks, cook them for 2 minutes each side for rare; 3 minutes for medium; and 4 minutes for well done. Keep turning the steaks throughout so they cook evenly. Remove from the pan and 'rest' on a warm plate covered in foil before cutting into 5mm/¼in thick slices.

5. Whisk the 3 tablespoons olive oil, balsamic vinegar, lemon juice and mustard to make a dressing and season with salt and pepper.

6. Arrange the rocket and tomatoes on 4 serving plates and top with the steak slices. Drizzle the dressing over the top and sprinkle with Parmesan shavings. Serve immediately with the swede chips.

OR YOU CAN TRY THIS...

⊙ Use parsnips or sweet potatoes instead of swede or mix some sautéed new potatoes into the salad.

⊙ Instead of making a dressing, just drizzle with balsamic vinegar and some lemon juice.

⊙ Use peppery watercress instead of rocket.

BEEF & PUMPKIN CASSEROLE

Slow-cooking brings out the flavour of food and makes meat really tender. This casserole can be made in advance and then cooled and frozen. You can also serve it with boiled rice, quinoa or gluten-free pasta.

SERVES 4
PREP: 15 MIN
COOK: 2–2½ HOURS

3 tbsp olive oil

2 celery stalks, diced

2 large carrots, sliced

400g/14oz pumpkin, peeled and cubed

500g/1lb 2oz lean chuck or braising steak or topside, all visible fat removed, cubed

750ml/26fl oz (generous 3 cups) onion-free beef stock

1 x 400g/14oz can tomatoes

2 tbsp tomato paste

grated zest and juice of 1 orange

1 tbsp balsamic vinegar

1 bay leaf

1–2 tbsp cornflour (cornstarch), (optional)

salt and freshly ground black pepper

a handful of parsley, finely chopped, to sprinkle

baked or mashed potatoes, to serve

1. Preheat the oven to 170°C, 325°F, gas mark 3.

2. Heat the oil in a large flameproof casserole, set over a low heat. Add the celery, carrots and pumpkin and cook for 8–10 minutes, stirring occasionally, until tender. Remove the vegetables and set on one side.

3. Add the beef to the casserole and cook over a medium heat for about 5 minutes, stirring often, until browned and seared all over. Add the beef stock, tomatoes and tomato paste, stirring all the time. Bring to the boil and remove from the heat.

4. Return the vegetables to the casserole, together with the orange zest and juice, balsamic vinegar and bay leaf. Cover with a lid and cook in the preheated oven for 1½–2 hours or until the beef is really tender, the vegetables are cooked and the liquid has reduced. You can thicken it if required by mixing some cornflour with a little cold water to make a paste and stirring it into the casserole.

5. Discard the bay leaf and season to taste with salt and pepper. Serve immediately, sprinkled with parsley with baked or mashed potatoes.

OR YOU CAN TRY THIS...
- Add a few drops of Worcestershire or soy sauce instead of balsamic vinegar.
- Substitute swede for the pumpkin.

TIP
Check the casserole after an hour to see if it needs some more liquid – don't let it dry out.

CHILLI CON CARNE WITH QUINOA

You can make this quick chilli a day in advance and keep it covered in the fridge overnight, ready to reheat for supper the following day. It also freezes well.

SERVES 4
PREP: 10 MIN
COOK: 50 MIN

1 tbsp olive oil

2 celery stalks, diced

2 carrots, diced

1 red chilli, finely diced

500g/1lb 2oz (2¼ cups) minced (ground) beef (max. 5% fat)

1 tbsp cumin seeds

1 tsp ground cinnamon

1 tsp chipotle paste or chilli powder

2 x 400g/14oz cans chopped tomatoes

300ml/10½fl oz (1¼ cups) onion-free beef stock

85g/3oz canned chickpeas, rinsed and drained

180g/6oz (1 cup) quinoa

1 small ripe avocado, peeled, stoned (pitted) and diced

juice of 1 lime

a handful of coriander (cilantro), roughly chopped

salt and freshly ground black pepper

4 tbsp plain or lactose-free yoghurt, to serve

1. Heat the oil in a large saucepan and cook the celery, carrots and chilli, stirring occasionally, over a low to medium heat for about 8–10 minutes until softened.

2. Add the beef, cumin seeds, cinnamon and chipotle paste or chilli powder. Cook for 5 minutes, stirring occasionally, until the beef is browned all over.

3. Add the tomatoes and stock and simmer gently for 25–30 minutes until the sauce reduces and thickens. Stir in the chickpeas and cook for 5 minutes to warm them through. Season to taste with salt and pepper.

4. Meanwhile, cook the quinoa according to the instructions on the packet.

5. Serve the chilli on a bed of quinoa and scatter the avocado tossed in the lime juice and coriander over the top. Add a spoonful of yoghurt to each serving.

OR YOU CAN TRY THIS…

- Serve with boiled or steamed rice or corn tortillas heated on a hot griddle.

- Try minced chicken instead of beef.

- You can also add diced sweet potato, peppers and aubergine (eggplant).

KOFTAS ON GREEN HERBS
WITH TOMATO RICE

For this North African dish, spiced minced meat – usually lamb, but sometimes beef or a mixture of both – is packed cylindrically around skewers, then grilled to a crust. The koftas are served on a bed of herbs and accompanied by tasty tomato-flavoured rice.

SERVES 4
PREP: 20 MIN
COOK: ABOUT 25 MIN
FREEZING: Not suitable

575g/1¼lb finely minced (ground) lamb

1 tsp ground allspice

6 fresh mint leaves, finely shredded, or 1 tsp dried mint

salt and freshly ground black pepper

olive oil, for brushing

FOR THE TOMATO RICE
2 tbsp garlic-infused olive oil

225g/8oz long-grain rice

200g/7oz can peeled plum tomatoes

TO SERVE
5 spring onions (scallions), green parts only, finely chopped

3 tbsp chopped parsley

2 tbsp chopped mint

lemon wedges

parsley sprigs

⊙ ⊙ ⊙

KOFTAS ON GREEN HERBS

1. First prepare the tomato rice. Heat the garlic oil in a heavy-based saucepan (which has a close-fitting lid). Add the rice and stir over the heat for 1 minute until is glossy.

2. Tip the can of tomatoes into a sieve over the saucepan and press through, then fill the can with cold water and pour that in too. Bring to the boil and season with salt and pepper. Cover with a tight-fitting lid, turn the heat down as low as possible and simmer for 10 minutes.

3. Line the grill rack with foil and preheat the grill. Put the minced lamb into a bowl and sprinkle in the allspice, mint and plenty of salt and pepper. Use your hands to mix together thoroughly to a paste. Divide into 8 portions and mould each into a sausage shape around a skewer. Brush them all over with olive oil.

4. When the rice has simmered for 10 minutes, turn off heat without removing lid, and leave for a further 12–15 minutes.

5. In the meantime, arrange the meat skewers on the lined grill pan and grill, turning regularly, for about 10–12 minutes until well browned all over.

6. Meanwhile, mix the spring onion greens with the parsley and mint and spread in a layer on one side of each serving plate. Lay the koftas on top.

7. Fork up the rice gently, correct the seasoning and serve with the koftas. Garnish with lemon wedges and parsley sprigs.

NOTE: If wooden skewers are used, soak them in cold water for at least 10 minutes before packing the meat around them. This prevents exposed tips from burning during grilling.

MOROCCAN LAMB TAGINE

Raisins add sweetness to this spicy stew, rather than the traditional dates, apricots or prunes. It is sprinkled with pomegranate seeds, which contain moderate amounts of fructan and are allowed in small quantities.

SERVES 4
PREP: 15 MIN
COOK: 45–55 MIN

2 tbsp olive oil

500g/1lb 2oz lean leg of lamb or lamb fillet, cubed

1 red (bell) pepper, deseeded and sliced

1 large aubergine (eggplant), cubed

2 courgettes (zucchini), cut into chunks

1 tsp ground cumin

½ tsp ground ginger

1 tbsp ras el hanout spice mix

300ml/10½fl oz (1¼ cups) hot onion-free chicken stock

a few strands of saffron

chopped pulp and zest of 1 preserved lemon

4 juicy tomatoes, chopped

85g/3oz (½ cup) raisins

85g/3oz (½ cup) canned chickpeas, rinsed and drained

4 tbsp purple or black olives, stoned (pitted)

a dash of lemon juice (optional)

salt and freshly ground black pepper

a handful of coriander (cilantro), chopped

a handful of flat-leaf parsley, chopped

a dash of harissa

110g/4oz (½ cup) natural yoghurt or lactose-free yoghurt

seeds from ½ small pomegranate

cooked quinoa, to serve

○ ○ ○

...MOROCCAN LAMB TAGINE

1. Heat the oil in a heavy-bottomed pan and add the lamb, cook over a medium to high heat, turning it occasionally, for 5 minutes until browned all over. Remove and set aside.

2. Add the red pepper, aubergine and courgettes and cook for 4–5 minutes until softened. Stir in the ground spices and cook for 1 minute. Add the hot stock, saffron, preserved lemon, tomatoes and raisins. Return the lamb to the pan and arrange on top of the vegetables.

3. Cover with a tight-fitting lid and cook gently over a low heat for 30–40 minutes, until the lamb is cooked and the liquid has reduced.

4. Stir in the chickpeas, olives and lemon juice (if using). Season to taste and simmer gently, uncovered, for 5 minutes. Add the coriander (cilantro) and parsley.

5. Swirl the harissa into the yoghurt in a small serving bowl. Then serve the tagine, sprinkled with pomegranate seeds, with the quinoa. Place the yoghurt on the side for spooning over as you wish..

OR YOU CAN TRY THIS...

- Serve the tagine with brown rice instead of quinoa.

- Use chicken thighs instead of lamb.

- If you can't get preserved lemons, coarsely chop a fresh one and add to the tagine.

- For extra heat, stir a blob of fiery-red harissa paste into the tagine at the end.

ROAST STUFFED TURKEY

This roasting method ensures that the bird remains moist and the skin beautifully brown and crisp. Try to use a fresh rather than a defrosted frozen turkey – the flavour is much better, and less water emerges during cooking. Free-range bronze turkeys are particularly flavoursome.

SERVES 8 (PLUS LEFTOVERS)
PREP: 45 MIN
COOK: 3½-5 HOURS, PLUS RESTING

4.5–5.5kg/10–12lb turkey, with giblets
180–225g/6–8oz (¾–1 cup butter), softened
salt and freshly ground black pepper

FOR THE CRANBERRY & ORANGE STUFFING:
1 tbsp garlic-infused olive oil, plus extra to drizzle
75g/2½oz cubed pancetta
250g/9oz (1½ cups) minced (ground) pork
150g/5oz (scant 3 cups) fresh gluten-free breadcrumbs
2 eggs
75g/2½oz dried cranberries
zest of 2 large oranges
2 tbsp toasted pine nuts, roughly chopped
30g/1oz chopped fresh soft herbs, e.g. parsley, thyme,
    oregano, chives, basil

FOR THE GRAVY:
1 carrot, peeled and chopped
a few parsley sprigs
1 bay leaf
a few black peppercorns
1 tbsp cornflour (cornstarch)

⊙ ⊙ ⊙

...ROAST STUFFED TURKEY

1. Preheat the oven to 180°C, 350°F, gas mark 4. Remove the giblets from turkey, discard the liver and put aside the rest to make stock for gravy. Wash the bird thoroughly inside and out; dry with kitchen paper. Spread butter over the turkey and season well. Weigh bird and calculate cooking time: allow 20 minutes per 450 g/1lb, plus 20 minutes extra.

2. Line a large roasting tin (pan) with foil, bringing the edges over the rim. Place the turkey in the centre, covering it loosely with another sheet of foil, tucking the edges inside the rim. Roast for the calculated cooking time, removing the cover foil for the last 30 minutes to brown the turkey. Test the deepest part of each thigh with a skewer to check that the juices run clear and the bird is cooked through. Transfer to a platter, cover and rest in a warm place for 15 minutes.

3. While the turkey is cooking, prepare the stock for the gravy. Place the reserved giblets in a saucepan with the carrot, parsley, bay leaf and peppercorns. Cover with at least 600ml/1 pint (2½ cups) water, bring to the boil, then simmer for 1 hour. Strain.

4. To prepare the stuffing, heat the oil in a small frying pan and fry the pancetta until golden and crisp. Transfer the pancetta and it's flavoured oil to a bowl and add all the remaining stuffing ingredients. Mix everything together well and season to taste with salt and pepper. Roll the mixture into 16 balls and place them in a small, greased baking tray. Drizzle a little more garlic oil over the top. Bake them in the oven with the turkey for the last 25 minutes of cooking, turning once halfway through, until golden and cooked through.

5. Skim off the fat from the turkey roasting juices, reserving 3 tablespoons. Add the juices to the gravy stock. Heat the reserved fat in a saucepan and stir in the cornflour. Whisk in the stock and bring to the boil. Simmer for 5 minutes, season and strain into a warm sauceboat.

6. Serve the turkey with the stuffing, gravy and traditional accompaniments.

SPRING CHICKEN & HERB CASSEROLE

Cooking the whole chicken in the broth gives this casserole a lovely rich flavour. It is packed with baby spring vegetables and perked up at the end with handfuls of herbs and lemon zest, making it a great light alternative to a heavier Sunday roast. Ask your butcher to joint the chicken for you if you're not sure, but make sure you get the carcass back, too.

SERVES 4
PREP: 30 MIN
COOK: 45 MIN

350ml/12fl oz (1½ cups) white wine

1 bouquet garni

1 corn-fed or free-range chicken, weighing about 1.4kg/3 lb, jointed into 8 pieces

2 tbsp garlic-infused olive oil

30g/1oz (2 tbsp) butter

250g/9oz chantenay carrots, halved if large

450g/1lb baby new potatoes

2 celery stalks, cut into 5cm/2in lengths

600ml/1 pint (2½ cups) onion-free chicken stock

1 tbsp cornflour (cornstarch)

150g/5oz sliced spring greens

2 large handfuls of fresh soft herbs, e.g. basil, tarragon, thyme, chives, parsley, roughly chopped

grated zest and juice of 1 lemon

salt and freshly ground black pepper

1. Pour the wine into a saucepan and add the bouquet garni. Bring to the boil and simmer until reduced by half. Allow to cool, then remove and discard the bouquet garni.

2. Season the chicken pieces. Heat half of the oil and butter in a large frying pan, add half the chicken joints and brown all over, then transfer to a flameproof casserole. Repeat with a little more oil and butter and the remaining joints.

3. Put the carrots, potatoes and celery into the casserole and pour over the reduced white wine, along with the stock. Bring to the boil, lower the heat, cover and simmer very slowly for 30 minutes until the meat and vegetables are cooked through and tender. You may need to stir it carefully a couple of times throughout cooking to make sure things aren't drying out on top.

4. Remove the chicken and vegetables with a slotted spoon and transfer them to a warmed serving dish. Mix the cornflour with a little water in a bowl and add it to the stock in the pan. Raise the heat a little and allow it to bubble and begin to thicken a little. Add the spring greens and let them cook in the liquid as it thickens.

5. Once the greens are tender and the sauce thickened and rich, stir in the herbs and lemon zest and juice. Taste and adjust the seasoning. Pour the sauce over the chicken and vegetables and mix gently to combine, then serve.

TUNISIAN SPICED LAMB WITH QUINOA SALAD

We have used ground spices for convenience, but you can make a more authentic dish by dry-frying coriander and cumin seeds for 2 minutes, then grinding them to a powder.

SERVES 4
PREP: 20 MIN
COOK: 15 MIN

250g/9oz (1½ cups) quinoa

16 small black olives, stoned (pitted)

200g/7oz baby plum tomatoes, quartered

1 baby avocado, stoned (pitted), peeled and diced

85g/3oz feta cheese, diced

a handful of mint, chopped

1 tsp ground coriander

1 tsp ground cumin

a pinch of ground cinnamon

4 lean lamb steaks, all visible fat removed

1 tbsp olive oil

salt and freshly ground black pepper

a handful of wild rocket (arugula), to serve

○ ○ ◎

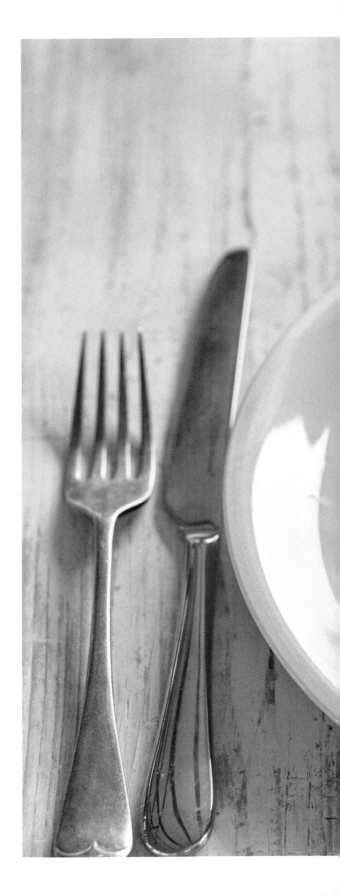

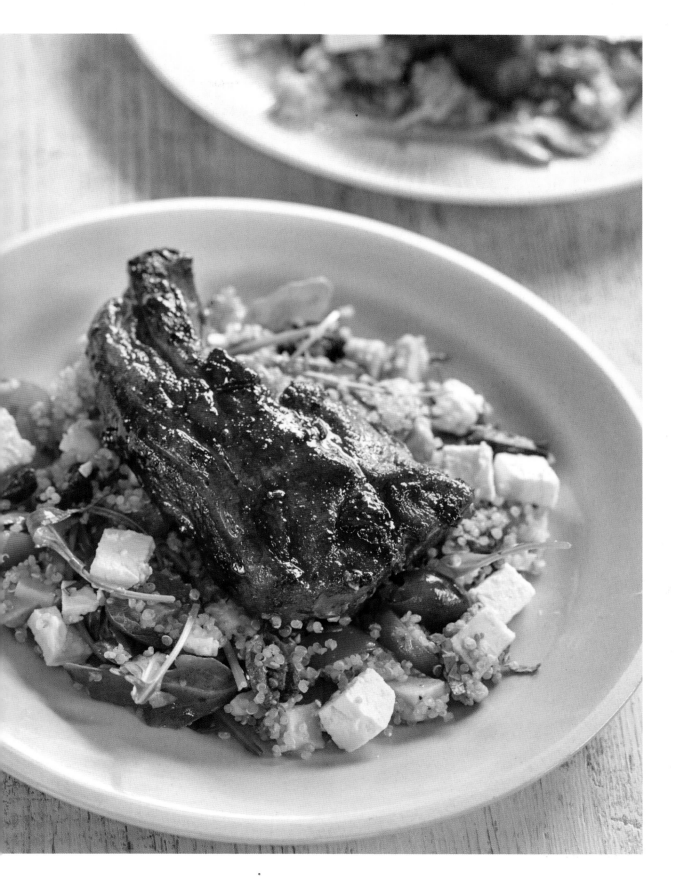

... TUNISIAN SPICED LAMB

FOR THE LEMON DRESSING:

3 tbsp fruity olive oil

1 tbsp white wine or apple cider vinegar

grated zest and juice of 1 large lemon

1 tsp Dijon mustard

a dash of lemon juice (optional)

a handful of coriander (cilantro), chopped

a handful of flat-leaf parsley, chopped

seeds from ½ small pomegranate

a dash of harissa

110g/4oz (½ cup) natural yoghurt or lactose-free yoghurt

1. Cook the quinoa in a pan of boiling water, according to the manufacturer's instructions on the packet. Drain well.

2. Make the lemon dressing: mix all the ingredients together in a small bowl or shake in a screwtop jar. Season with salt and pepper.

3. Put the hot quinoa in a bowl with the olives, tomatoes, avocado, feta and mint. Add most of the lemon dressing and toss together gently. Set aside.

4. Rub the ground spices and a little ground black pepper into both sides of the lamb steaks. Lightly brush a ridged griddle pan with oil and set over a medium to high heat. Add the lamb to the hot pan and cook for 3–5 minutes each side, depending on how pink or well cooked you like it.

5. Slice the steaks into 1–2.5cm/½–1in thick strips and arrange them on top of the quinoa salad on 4 serving plates. Add the rocket leaves and drizzle with them with the remaining dressing.

OR YOU CAN TRY THIS...

- Use chopped parsley or coriander (cilantro) instead of mint.

- Add some crushed caraway seeds to the spice mixture.

- Make it hotter by adding crushed chilli (hot pepper) flakes or serving the lamb with harissa.

SPICY PORK BURGERS
WITH STIR-FRIED KALE

Everybody loves burgers and these pork ones, enhanced with Thai flavourings, are unusual and delicious. They taste equally good served with stir-fried vegetables from your FODMAP food list.

SERVES 4
PREP: 15 MIN
COOK: 20 MIN

450g/1lb lean pork fillet/tenderloin, all visible fat removed

1 red chilli, deseeded and diced

1 stalk lemongrass, peeled and finely sliced

1 tsp grated fresh root ginger

2 tsp nam pla (Thai fish sauce)

grated zest and juice of ½ lime

a handful of coriander (cilantro), finely chopped

salt and freshly ground black pepper

boiled rice, to serve

sweet chilli sauce, for drizzling

FOR THE STIR-FRIED KALE:

1 tbsp coconut oil or sunflower oil

1 tsp black mustard seeds

2.5cm/1in piece fresh root ginger, peeled and diced

400g/14oz kale, coarsely shredded

3–4 tbsp 0% fat Greek yoghurt or lactose-free yoghurt

1. Blitz the pork, chilli, lemongrass, ginger, nam pla, lime zest and juice and coriander in a food processor or blender. Season with a little salt and pepper.

2. Divide the mixture into 4 large or 8 small portions, and, using your hands, mould each one into a burger shape.

3. Cook the burgers under a preheated hot grill (broiler) for 6–8 minutes each side, until golden brown and the pork is cooked right through and no longer pink.

4. Meanwhile, cook the kale: heat the oil in a wok or deep frying pan (skillet) over a medium heat and cook the mustard seeds and ginger for 1 minute until the seeds pop and release their aroma. Add the kale and stir-fry for 2–3 minutes until just tender. Off the heat, stir in the yoghurt.

5. Serve the burgers and stir-fried kale with some boiled rice, drizzled with chilli sauce.

OR YOU CAN TRY THIS...

⊙ Use soy sauce instead of nam pla.

⊙ Make the burgers with minced beef or chicken instead of pork.

⊙ Squeeze a lime over the cooked burgers.

⊙ Serve the burgers in gluten-free rolls or wraps with salad and lactose-free yoghurt.

PORK & ROOTS CASSEROLE

This traditional dish is all about getting back to basics and enjoying really flavoursome food. It makes a wonderfully warming supper on a cold day.

SERVES 4
PREP: 15 MIN
COOK: 1¾ HOURS

2 tbsp olive oil

4 x 150g/5oz lean pork steaks

2 celery stalks, diced

2 carrots, cut into chunks

3 parsnips, peeled and cut into wedges

400g/14oz potatoes, peeled and cut into wedges

400ml/14fl oz (1¾ cups) onion-free chicken stock

240ml/8fl oz (1 cup) dry white wine

1 tbsp whole-grain Dijon mustard

2 bay leaves

1 tbsp chopped fresh sage

1 strip orange zest

1–2 tbsp cornflour (cornstarch)

4 tbsp crème fraîche

salt and freshly ground black pepper

2 tbsp finely chopped parsley, to sprinkle

steamed green beans, to serve

1. Preheat the oven to 170°C, 325°F, gas mark 3.

2. Heat the oil in a flameproof casserole dish. Add the port and cook the pork over a medium to high heat for about 5 minutes until browned on both sides. Remove from the pan and set aside.

3. Add the celery, carrots, parsnips and potatoes to the casserole and cook for about 5 minutes until slightly softened. Add the browned pork and pour in the chicken stock and white wine. Bring to the boil, then stir in the mustard, herbs and orange zest. Season with salt and pepper.

4. Cover the casserole with a lid and cook in the preheated oven for 1½ hours until the pork and vegetables are cooked and the liquid has reduced.

5. Blend the cornflour with a little water to make a smooth paste and add to the casserole. Put it on the hob over a low heat and stir with a wooden spoon until the sauce thickens. Stir in the crème fraîche.

6. Spoon the pork and vegetables in their sauce onto 4 serving plates and sprinkle with parsley. Serve with green beans.

OR YOU CAN TRY THIS...

- Use chunks of lean pork leg or shoulder instead of steaks.

- The casserole works well with chicken thighs. Cook in the same way as the pork.

- Vary the root vegetables: try swede (rutabaga) or celeriac (celery root).

- For a hint of sweet aniseed, add some fennel wedges.

- Season with a dash of Worcestershire sauce and some paprika.

SMOKEY CHICKEN FAJITAS

You can serve this delicious Mexican dish with tortillas, a little guacamole and some thick Greek yoghurt. Do make sure that your tortillas are cornmeal ones, and not made with wheat.

SERVES 6
PREP: 30 MIN, PLUS MARINATING
COOK: 25 MIN

2–3 hot chillies, deseeded (if wished) and thinly sliced, plus extra to serve

2 tbsp garlic-infused olive oil, plus extra for frying

2 tsp sweet smoked paprika, plus extra if needed

4 chicken breast fillets, skinned and cut into strips

2 large aubergines (eggplants)

4 red, yellow or orange (bell) peppers (or a mixture), deseeded and cut into thin strips

8 spring onions (scallions), green parts only, cut into strips

salt and freshly ground black pepper

18 small corn tortillas, to serve

thick Greek yogurt, to serve

FOR THE GUACAMOLE:

1½ avocados, peeled and diced

1 beef tomato, deseeded and diced

a handful of coriander (cilantro) leaves, chopped, plus extra sprigs to serve

zest of 2 limes and juice of 1

⊙ ⊙ ⊙

···SMOKEY CHICKEN FAJITAS

1. Combine the chillies, garlic-infused oil, smoked paprika and chicken in a shallow dish. Season generously with salt and pepper, stir well, cover and leave to marinate in a cool place for at least 1 hour or overnight.

2. Cook the aubergines directly over a gas hob, turning regularly so that all parts of the vegetable are exposed to the flames and the skins blacken and bubble. To cook through, they will take about 15 minutes, depending on the size of the aubergines. They should feel soft throughout. Set aside until cool enough to handle, then peel away the skins and chop the flesh into strips (it should be very soft).

3. Meanwhile make the guacamole: combine all the ingredients in a small bowl and season with salt and pepper. Set aside.

4. Heat a little more oil in a large frying pan (skillet) or wok and add the marinated chicken and chillies. Cook, stirring, over a high heat until thoroughly browned on the outside. Remove the chicken from the pan. Add the peppers to the pan and cook, stirring, over a high heat for about 5 minutes until the peppers are softened, then add the spring onion greens and cook for 2 minutes until they are tender, but still green.

5. Return the chicken to the pan, lower the heat and cook everything together for about 5 minutes, stirring occasionally, or until the chicken is cooked right through. Stir in the aubergine strips, taste and season, and add a little more smoked paprika, if wished.

6. Meanwhile, warm the tortillas in a dry frying pan, keeping them warm in a clean tea towel as you go. (It's easiest to have a couple of frying pans on the go for this.)

7. Transfer the chicken mix to a serving bowl and sprinkle with coriander sprigs. Serve alongside the tortillas, guacamole and Greek yogurt, for people to assemble their own fajitas.

SPEEDY SWEET & SOUR PORK

This is a speedy and healthy FODMAP version of a classic dish. It's as quick to make at home from scratch as it is to order and wait for a take-away!

SERVES 4
PREP: 15 MIN
COOK: 15 MIN

225g/8oz (1 cup) basmati rice (dry weight)

2 tbsp sunflower or groundnut (peanut) oil

450g/1lb lean pork fillet, cut into thin strips

2.5cm/1in piece fresh root ginger, peeled and finely diced

1 green (bell) pepper, deseeded and cut into chunks

1 red (bell) pepper, deseeded and cut into chunks

2 carrots, peeled and cut into thin matchsticks

4 pineapple rings, canned in natural juice, cut into chunks

salt and freshly ground black pepper

FOR THE SWEET AND SOUR SAUCE:
3 tbsp mirin or white wine vinegar

4 tbsp light soy sauce

1 tbsp tomato paste or ketchup

180ml/6fl oz (¾ cup) fresh orange juice

2 tsp brown sugar

2 tbsp cornflour (cornstarch)

1. Make the sweet and sour sauce: mix all the ingredients together in a bowl until smooth and the cornflour is thoroughly blended.

2. Cook the rice according to the instructions on the packet.

3. Meanwhile, heat the oil in a wok or deep frying pan (skillet) set over a high heat. When it is very hot and the oil is smoking, add the pork and stir-fry for 5 minutes, until golden brown and cooked through. Add the ginger, peppers and carrots and stir-fry for 2–3 minutes.

4. Add the pineapple and pour in the sweet and sour sauce mixture. Reduce the heat and stir for 1 minute, until the sauce thickens and coats the pork and vegetables.

5. Check the seasoning and serve immediately with the boiled rice.

OR YOU CAN TRY THIS...

⊙ Use cubed chicken breast instead of pork.

⊙ Sprinkle with chopped coriander (cilantro) or chives before serving.

⊙ Serve with some stir-fried crisp shredded Chinese leaves (Chinese cabbage).

DOUGH RECIPES

The following two basic gluten-free dough recipes are great to have up your sleeve, as they can be easily adapted to form the base of lots of delicious dishes, from calzone to a classic savoury pie.

PIZZA DOUGH

Use this low-FODMAP pizza dough recipe to create quick and easy meals that you can dapt easily for the whole family. Make the rocket and prosciutto pizza on page 162, be inspired by the suggestions below, or go completely off-piste with your own flavour combos!

**MAKES ENOUGH FOR
   4 X 25CM/10IN PIZZAS
PREP: 20 MIN**

400g/14oz gluten-free flour

1 tsp salt

1 x 7g/¼oz sachet fast-action
   dried yeast

1 tsp sugar

1 tbsp chopped rosemary

3 tbsp olive oil

240ml/8fl oz (1 cup) warm water

1. Put the flour, salt, yeast, sugar, rosemary and olive oil in a food processor and blitz until thoroughly mixed. Add the water in a trickle through the feed tube until you have a smooth, soft dough. If it's too dry, add a little more water; too sticky, add some more flour.

2. Turn the dough out onto a work surface, lightly dusted with flour, and knead with your hands until it's really smooth. Divide into 4 equal-sized pieces and roll out each one out to a 25cm/10in circle. Cover with toppings as per the recipe or your own choosing.

3. Cook and oven preheated to 220°C, 425°F, gas mark 7, for about 10–15 minutes until the bases are golden and crisp and the cheese has melted.

OR YOU CAN TRY THIS...

⊙ Spike the tomato pizza sauce with hot smoked paprika and sprinkle over sliced jarred roasted red (bell) peppers and jalapeno peppers.

⊙ For a classic Fiorentina, cover the base with tomato sauce, then wilted spinach. Crack an egg in the middle and sprinkle with planty of grated Parmesan and a little grated nutmeg.

PASTRY DOUGH

It's great to have a good gluten-free pastry recipe in your arsenal, to use for quiches, tarts and pies. Use this basic recipe to make the Cheesy Tomato and Bacon Quiche overleaf, or experiment, adding your own low-FODMAP fillings (see suggestions below).

**MAKES ENOUGH FOR A
   23CM/9IN TART OR QUICHE
PREP: 20 MIN**

150g/5oz (1 cup) rice flour, plus
   extra for dusting

50g/2oz (½ cup) polenta
   (cornmeal)

1 tsp xanthan gum

a pinch of salt

100g/4oz (½ cup) butter, diced,
   plus extra for greasing

1 medium free-range egg, beaten

1. Put the rice flour, polenta, xanthan gum and a pinch of salt in a large mixing bowl. Add the butter and rub in with your fingertips until the mixture resembles fine breadcrumbs. Stir in the beaten egg and 1 tablespoon of cold water (if required) until you have a soft dough. Form into a ball, then chill until needed.

OR YOU CAN TRY THIS…

⊙ Cooked shredded chicken, a few mushrooms (browned in a frying pan), and tarragon.

⊙ Chunks of hot smoked salmon, wilted spinach, lemon zest and dill.

⊙ Griddled courgette (zucchini), crumbled feta cheese and mint leaves.

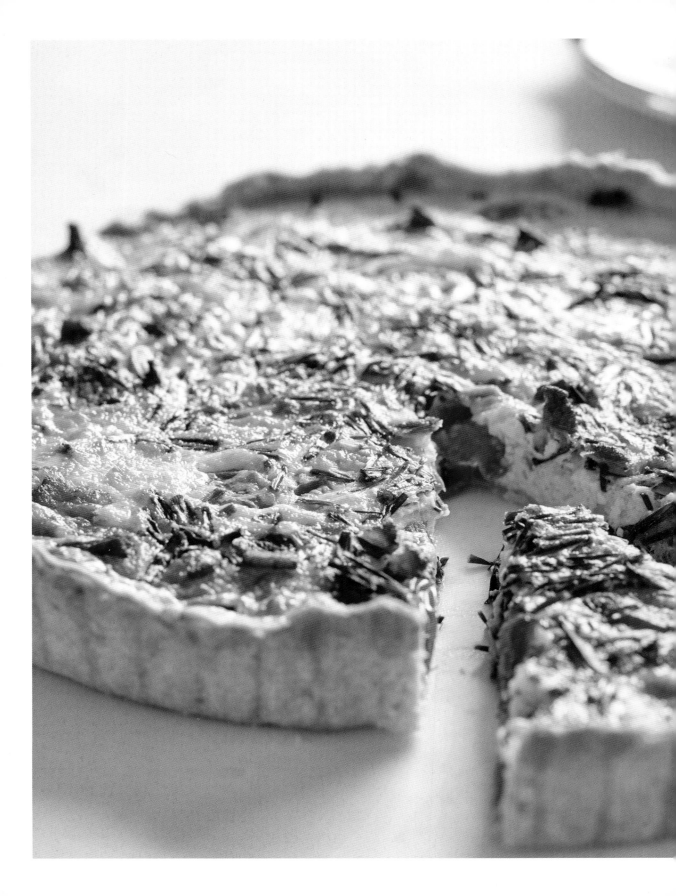

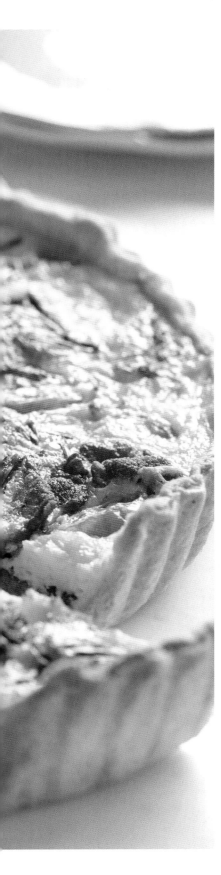

CHEESY TOMATO & BACON QUICHE

A delicious back to basics quiche made with gluten-free pastry (pie crust).

SERVES 4
PREP: 40 MIN
COOK: 1 HOUR

1 recipe quantity pastry dough
  (see page 157)

110g/4oz smoked streaky bacon,
  diced

150g/5oz baby plum tomatoes,
  halved

200g/7oz (2 cups) grated
  Cheddar cheese

4 medium free-range eggs

120ml/4fl oz (½ cup)
  semi-skimmed milk or
  lactose-free milk

180ml/6fl oz (¾ cup) double
  (heavy) lactose-free cream

a handful of chives, snipped

salt and freshly ground black
  pepper

salad, to serve

◎ ◎ ◎

... CHEESY TOMATO & BACON QUICHE

1. Preheat the oven to 190°C, 375°F, gas mark 5. Lightly butter a deep loose-bottomed (springform) 23cm/9in tart tin (pan).

2. Roll out the pastry dough on a lightly floured surface and use to line the tart tin. Trim the edges and prick the base with a fork. Place on a baking (cookie) sheet and chill in the fridge for 15 minutes.

3. Line the pastry in the tart tin with a piece of baking parchment (waxed paper) and fill with baking beans or raw uncooked rice. Bake 'blind' in the preheated oven for 15 minutes, then remove the paper and beans or rice and bake for 5 more minutes. Remove from the oven and lower the temperature to 170°C, 325°F, gas mark 3.

4. While the pastry is cooking, dry-fry the bacon in a small frying pan (skillet) for 3–4 minutes until crisp and golden. Drain on kitchen paper (towels).

5. Arrange the tomatoes in the pastry case the tart tin and sprinkle with the grated cheese. Scatter the bacon over the top.

6. Whisk the eggs, milk and cream in a large jug. Stir in the chives and some salt and pepper, to taste. Pour into the pastry case and bake in the oven for 30–40 minutes until the filling is set and golden brown on top.

7. Serve the quiche warm or cold, cut into slices with some salad.

OR YOU CAN TRY THIS...

- Vary the herbs – try parsley, basil or oregano.

- Use grated Swiss cheese or mix the Cheddar with some Parmesan.

- Try diced cooked ham instead of bacon or leave it out for a vegetarian version.

GAMMON, SPINACH & POTATO STACKS

This is an economical and homely supper that all the family will enjoy. If you have leftover cooked vegetables from a Sunday roast or previous meal, you can also mash them up and cook as below. A mixture of potatoes, swede (rutabaga), parsnips, carrots and green vegetables can be used instead of just the potatoes and spinach.

SERVES 4
PREP: 15 MIN
COOK: 30 MIN

450g/1lb potatoes, peeled and cut into chunks

250g/9oz baby spinach leaves

60g/2oz (¼ cup) half-fat crème fraîche or lactose-free yoghurt

1 bunch of chives, snipped

1 tsp sweet smoked paprika

1 tbsp olive oil

4 lean gammon steaks, all visible fat removed

4 medium free-range eggs

salt and freshly ground black pepper

mustard, tomato ketchup or spicy chutney, to serve

1. Bring the potatoes to the boil in a large pan of lightly salted water. Reduce the heat to a simmer and cook for 10–15 minutes until tender but not mushy. Drain well.

2. Put the spinach in a colander and pour boiling water over it. Press down with a saucer to squeeze out any excess liquid. Allow to cool a little and chop it finely.

3. Mash the potatoes with the crème fraîche. Stir in the spinach, chives, and paprika, and season to taste with salt and pepper. Divide the mashed potato into 4 portions and, with your hands, shape each one into a round 'cake'.

4. Heat the oil in a non-stick frying pan (skillet) over a low to medium heat and cook the potato cakes for 4–5 minutes each side, until golden brown. Remove from the pan and keep warm.

5. Meanwhile, cook the gammon steaks under a preheated hot grill (broiler) for about 4–5 minutes each side.

6. Break the eggs into a pan of simmering water and cook for about 3 minutes, until the whites are set but the yolks are still runny.

7. Place a potato cake on each serving plate and cover with a gammon steak. Top with a poached egg and serve immediately with mustard, ketchup or chutney.

OR YOU CAN TRY THIS…

- Instead of gammon, use chicken breast fillets or lean fillet steaks.

- Vegetarians can use tofu instead.

ROCKET & PROSCIUTTO PIZZAS

If wished, you can make the tomato sauce a day in advance and keep it in an airtight jar or container in the fridge until you're ready to make and assemble the pizzas.

SERVES 4
PREP: 25 MIN
COOK: 25–30 MIN

1 recipe quantity pizza dough (see page 156)

FOR THE TOMATO SAUCE:
3 tbsp olive oil

2 celery stalks, diced

1 x 400g/14oz can plum tomatoes, chopped

2 tbsp tomato paste

a pinch of sugar

salt and freshly ground black pepper

○ ○ ○

FOR THE ROCKET (ARUGULA) & PROSCIUTTO TOPPING:
350g/12oz mozzarella, torn into pieces or cut into cubes

a few basil leaves

olive oil, for drizzling

85g/3oz thinly sliced prosciutto or Parma ham, torn into strips

2 large handfuls of wild rocket (arugula)

balsamic vinegar, for drizzling

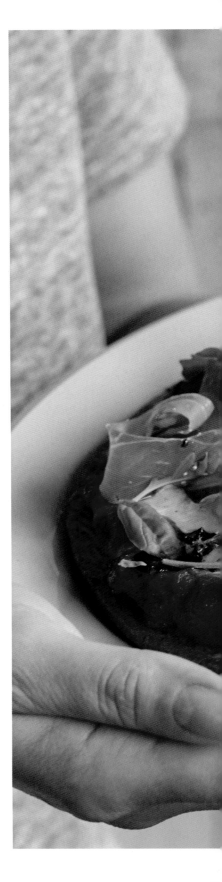

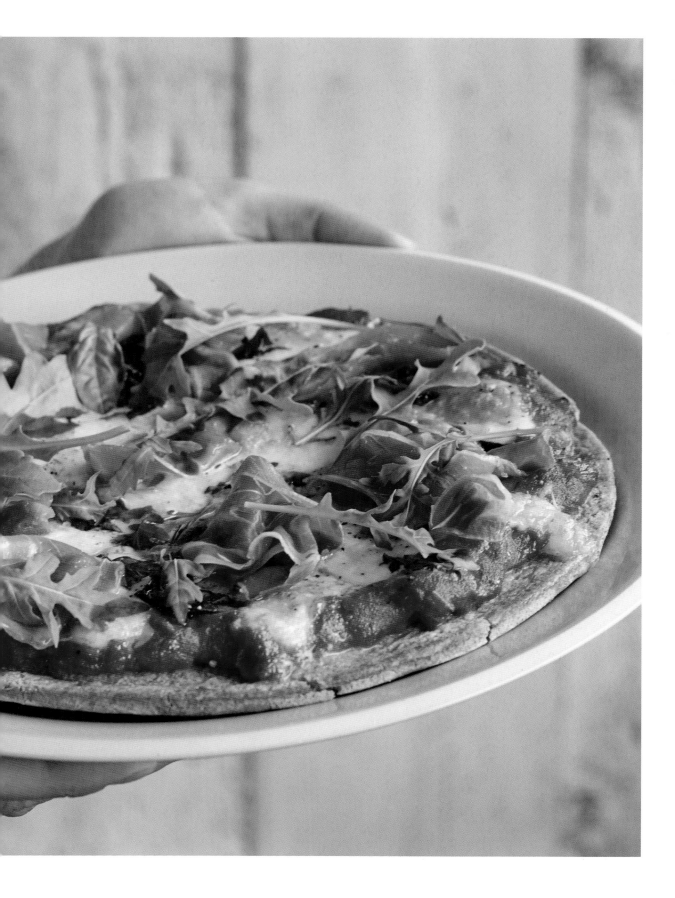

···ROCKET & PROSCIUTTO PIZZAS

1. Preheat the oven to 220°C, 425°F, gas mark 7.

2. Make the tomato sauce: heat the olive oil in a frying pan (skillet) set over a low heat, add the celery and cook, stirring occasionally, for about 5 minutes until softened. Add the tomatoes, tomato paste and sugar and simmer for 10 minutes or until reduced and thickened. Season with salt and pepper.

3. Divide the pizza dough into 4 equal-sized pieces and roll each one out to a 25cm/10in circle. Place these on baking (cookie) sheets and spread with the tomato sauce, leaving a thin border around the edge. Scatter the mozzarella and basil over the top and drizzle with olive oil. Set aside for 15 minutes.

4. Cook in the preheated oven for about 10–15 minutes until the bases are golden and crisp and the cheese has melted. Top with the prosciutto and rocket, drizzle with balsamic vinegar and serve immediately.

OR YOU CAN TRY THIS...

- ◎ Scatter the tomato sauce with some griddled sliced (bell) peppers or use bottled ones.

- ◎ Add some hot chilli (hot pepper) flakes to the tomato sauce.

- ◎ Use burrata instead of mozzarella.

- ◎ Break an egg into the centre of each pizza before cooking.

PAN-FRIED DUCK BREASTS WITH ROSTI & PORT & BLUEBERRY SAUCE

Rosy pink, tender slices of duck breast are served on golden parsnip and potato cakes and accompanied by a rich blueberry and Port sauce. If possible, buy the large French magrets – one of these easily serves two. Otherwise you will need four standard-sized duck breasts.

SERVES 4
PREP: 30 MIN
COOK: 20–25 MIN

2 large duck breast fillets, each about 350g/12oz, or
    4 medium duck breast fillets, at room temperature
salt and freshly ground black pepper
green vegetables, to serve

FOR THE ROSTI:
300g/10½oz floury potatoes (about 1 large potato)
200g/7oz parsnip (about 1 large parsnip)
2 fresh sage leaves, finely chopped
2 tbsp garlic-infused olive oil
30g/1oz (2 tbsp) butter

FOR THE PORT & BLUEBERRY SAUCE:
250g/9oz (2 cups) frozen blueberries
210ml/7fl oz (scant 1 cup) port
1 tbsp finely chopped rosemary
1 tbsp finely chopped thyme
1 tbsp Worcestershire sauce
1 tsp sugar

◉ ◉ ◉

...PAN FRIED DUCK BREASTS

1. First make the sauce, as this will benefit from sitting for a little while. Put the blueberries and port in a small pan and cook for 10–15 minutes until the fruit is breaking down and it starts to look syrupy. Add the herbs, Worcestershire sauce and sugar and continue to cook for 5 minutes, or until thickened and rich. Season to taste with salt and pepper and set aside.

2. Use a sharp knife to score through the skin side of the duck. Rub with salt and pepper. Leave at room temperature for 15 minutes.

3. Meanwhile, start to make the rösti: peel and finely grate the potato and parsnip. Squeeze out as much moisture as possible in a clean tea towel and place in a bowl. Add the sage and season well with salt and pepper.

4. Preheat a heavy flameproof casserole. Add the duck breasts skin-side down and cook over a medium heat for 7–10 minutes depending on size, without moving them; the fat that runs out will prevent them sticking. Turn the breasts over and cook for 3–4 minutes, depending on size, until cooked but still pink in the middle. Remove from the pan and leave them to rest under a pieve of kitchen foil while you fry the rosti.

5. Heat the oil and butter in a large non-stick frying pan over low to medium heat. Divide the rosti mixture into 4 and form them into rough patties. Place them in the pan and press down hard with a fish slice. Cook for about 4 minutes or until golden brown on the underside; turn over and cook for a few minutes on the other side until crisp and golden. Remove and drain on kitchen paper (towels).

6. While the rosti are cooking, gently reheat the port and blueberry sauce, if necessary.

7. To serve, place a rösti on each warmed serving plate. Slice the duck and arrange evenly on top of the rösti. Spoon on the sauce and serve immediately with some greens.

LAMB BIRYANI

Biryani is a spectacular celebratory Indian dish of curried meat — lamb in this instance — and saffron-flecked rice. Although this is a simplified version, it does still take time to prepare, but is well worth the effort.

SERVES 6
PREP: 30 MIN, PLUS SOAKING
COOK: 2 HOURS

450g/1lb (2½ cups) white basmati rice

1 tbsp salt

6cm/2½in piece fresh root ginger, peeled and roughly chopped

3 tbsp flaked almonds

1 tbsp ground coriander

2 tsp ground cumin

1 tsp ground fenugreek

1 tsp ground asafoetida

3 tbsp garlic-infused olive oil

4 tbsp ghee or vegetable oil

675g/1½lb boned leg or shoulder of lamb, cut into 2.5cm/1in cubes

1 cinnamon stick

6 green cardamoms

6 cloves

150ml/5fl oz (⅔ cup) lactose-free yoghurt

1 tsp cayenne pepper

freshly grated nutmeg

1 tsp saffron strands

a pinch of ground turmeric

40g/1½oz (3 tbsp) butter

TO SERVE:

hard-boiled eggs

sultanas (golden raisins)

toasted almonds

garam masala

coriander (cilantro) sprigs

1. Wash the rice in a sieve under cold running water until the water runs clear. Tip into a bowl, add the salt and enough water to cover. Leave to soak for about 1 hour.

2. Put the ginger, almonds, ground spices and garlic-infused oil in a food processor or blender and purée until smooth.

3. Heat half the ghee or vegetable oil in a large flameproof casserole. Add the lamb in 2 batches and brown over a high heat, adding the remaining ghee or oil for the second batch. Remove from the pan and set aside.

○ ○ ○

4. Add the ginger and spice paste to the pan and cook over a fairly high heat for about 5 minutes until the paste is golden brown, stirring all the time. Add the whole spices and cook for 2 minutes. Add the meat to the pan and stir to coat in the spices.

5. Lower the heat and gradually add the yoghurt, a spoonful at a time, stirring constantly. Add 250ml/9fl oz (1 cup) water, bring to a gentle simmer, cover and cook for about 1 hour or until the meat is tender, stirring occasionally to prevent it catching on the bottom of the pan. Season with salt, cayenne and nutmeg.

6. Meanwhile, preheat the oven to150°C, 300°F, gas mark 2. Put the saffron in a small bowl with the turmeric and 4 tablespoons warm water; leave to soak.

7. Drain the rice. Add to a large pan of boiling salted water, stir with a fork, then bring back to the boil and cook for about 5 minutes, or until almost cooked, but still a little firm. Drain thoroughly.

8. Once the lamb has cooked for an hour, pile the rice on top of the meat. Drizzle the saffron liquid across the rice and dot with the butter. Cover the casserole with a double thickness of foil, then the lid. Bake in the oven for 30 minutes.

9. To serve, transfer to a platter, fluff the rice carefully with a fork and garnish with the eggs, sultanas, almonds, garam masala and coriander.

SPAGHETTI WITH LAMB RAGU

A good ragu needs long, slow cooking. The sauce is reduced to a flavoursome concentrate and the meat become meltingly tender. Tossed with perfectly cooked spaghetti and freshly grated Parmesan cheese, this is real Italian comfort food, which is hard to beat.

SERVES 6
PREP: 25 MIN
COOK: 2½–3 HOURS

3 tbsp extra-virgin olive oil

2 tsp fennel seeds, lightly crushed

2 carrots, finely diced

2 celery stalks, finely diced

500g/1lb 2oz (2¼ cups) minced (ground) lamb

400ml/14fl oz (1¾ cups) red wine

3 tbsp chopped oregano

1 rosemary sprig

1 cinnamon stick

1 tbsp dark brown sugar

1 tbsp tomato paste

2 x 400g/14oz cans chopped tomatoes

400g/14 oz gluten-free spaghetti (dry weight)

5 tbsp freshly grated Parmesan cheese

salt and freshly ground black pepper

1. Heat the oil in a saucepan. Add the fennel seeds and cook for 1 minute, then add the carrot and celery and cook, stirring, for 4 minutes, until starting to soften.

2. Add the lamb to the pan and cook for about 7 minutes, breaking up the pieces with a wooden spoon, until browned. Increase the heat and stir in the wine. Let bubble for 4–5 minutes until the liquid has reduced by about half.

3. Add the oregano, rosemary sprig, cinnamon, brown sugar and tomato paste to the pan. Add the canned tomatoes and their juice, as well as 1 can of water. Bring to the boil and season lightly with salt and pepper. Cook, covered, on a very low heat for about 2 hours, stirring occasionally, until the lamb is meltingly tender. Remove and discard the cinnamon and rosemary. Adjust the seasoning to taste.

4. Just before serving, cook the spaghetti in a large pan of boiling salted water until *al dente* or according to packet instructions. Drain thoroughly.

5. To serve, toss the ragu with the pasta and about half of the grated Parmesan. Serve at once, sprinkled with the remaining Parmesan.

SUPPERS

=

FISH

CHINESE SALMON PARCELS

There are no smells and virtually no washing up when you cook fish this way. It's also very healthy and nutritious with a delicate flavour. If you prefer it more robust, you can add a chilli or some five-spice powder to the parcels or serve with sweet chilli sauce.

SERVES 4
PREP: 15 MIN
COOK: 15 MIN

180g/6oz baby carrots, halved lengthways

8 asparagus spears, cut into 2.5cm/1in lengths

2 pak choi (bok choy), thickly sliced

2.5cm/1in piece fresh root ginger, peeled and cut into matchsticks

4 star anise

4 x 110g/4oz skinned salmon fillets

a few chives, snipped

freshly ground black pepper

4 tbsp onion-free vegetable stock

2 tbsp light soy sauce

grated zest and juice of 1 lime

225g/8oz (1 cup) basmati rice (dry weight)

1. Preheat the oven to 190°C, 375°F, gas mark 5.

2. Divide the carrots and asparagus between 4 large squares of parchment paper (waxed paper), then add the pak choi, ginger and star anise. Place the salmon on top and sprinkle with the chives. Season with black pepper and drizzle over the stock, soy sauce, and lime zest and juice, distributing them evenly between the parcels.

3. Fold the paper over the salmon and vegetables, twisting the ends securely together to make 4 sealed parcels. Place them on a baking tray (cookie sheet).

4. Cook in the preheated oven for 15 minutes until the vegetables are tender and the salmon is cooked right through.

5. Meanwhile, cook the rice according to the instructions on the packet.

6. Divide the rice between 4 serving plates and spoon the vegetables and salmon over the top.

OR YOU CAN TRY THIS...

- Use teriyaki sauce and mirin instead of soy sauce.

- Add some matchstick courgettes (zucchini), diced celery, water chestnuts, fine green beans or shredded mangetout (snow peas) to the parcels.

- Thai basil or coriander (cilantro) can be substituted for chives.

SALMON, SPINACH & POTATO BAKE

This crisp golden bake is really healthy and nutritious – it's packed with vitamins and minerals. Salmon is a great source of omega-3 oils, which are beneficial for our cardiovascular health and cholesterol levels.

SERVES 4
PREP: 15 MIN
COOK: 50–60 MIN

500g/1lb 2oz potatoes, peeled

400g/14oz baby spinach leaves

450g/1lb skinned salmon fillets, cut into large chunks

15g/½oz (1 tbsp) butter

salt and freshly ground black pepper

FOR THE WHITE SAUCE:

4 tbsp cornflour (cornstarch)

600ml/1 pint (2½ cups) skimmed milk or lactose-free milk

110g/3½oz (scant ½ cup) virtually fat-free fromage frais

a pinch of ground nutmeg

grated zest of 1 lemon

a handful of dill, finely chopped

salt and freshly ground black pepper

TIP
Keep some frozen salmon fillets in the freezer for making this.

1. Preheat the oven to 200°C, 400°F, gas mark 6.

2. Cook the whole peeled potatoes in a pan of boiling salted water for 10–12 minutes until just tender but still firm and not falling apart. Drain and set aside to cool.

3. Put the spinach in a colander and pour some boiling water over it. Drain well, pressing out the excess water with a saucer. Spoon into a large ovenproof baking dish with the salmon.

4. Make the white sauce: blend the cornflour with a little of the milk to a smooth paste. Heat the remaining milk in a pan and when it starts to boil, reduce the heat and stir in the cornflour mixture. Cook gently, stirring with a wooden spoon, for 2–3 minutes until the sauce is thick and smooth. Off the heat, stir in the fromage frais, nutmeg, lemon zest, dill and seasoning. Pour over the salmon and spinach.

5. Thinly slice the cooled potatoes lengthwise and arrange in overlapping slices over the salmon and spinach mixture until it is completely covered. Dot the top with butter.

6. Bake in the preheated oven for 30–40 minutes until the salmon is cooked and the potatoes are golden brown and crisp.

OR YOU CAN TRY THIS...

- Use chopped parsley or even some chives instead of dill.

- Sprinkle with some grated Cheddar cheese before baking.

- White fish fillets, e.g. cod, and prawns (shrimp) also work well.

SALMON
WITH SPRING VEGETABLE BROTH

You can taste the spring in this beautiful scented broth! If possible make your own vegetable stock or buy a good ready-made one rather than using stock cubes or powder – it will taste so much better and fresher.

SERVES 4
PREP: 15 MIN
COOK: 25 MIN

3 tbsp olive oil

1 small fennel bulb, thinly sliced

150g/5oz Chantenay baby carrots, trimmed

200g/7oz baby new potatoes, halved

960ml/32fl oz (4 cups) onion-free vegetable stock

12 thin asparagus spears, cut into short lengths

150g/5oz baby spinach leaves

a small bunch of mint, chopped

4 thick salmon fillets

salt and freshly ground black pepper

FOR THE HERB MAYONNAISE:
4 tbsp mayonnaise

60g/2oz (¼ cup) low-fat natural yoghurt or lactose-free yoghurt

2 tsp green pesto

a few sprigs of basil, chopped

a few sprigs of mint, chopped

1. Make the herb mayonnaise: mix all the ingredients together in a bowl and set aside.

2. Heat 2 tablespoons of the olive oil in a large saucepan over a low heat , add the fennel and carrots and cook for 5 minutes. Add the potatoes and cook for a further 5 minutes. Pour in the stock and bring to the boil.

3. Reduce the heat to a simmer and cook gently for 5 minutes. Add the asparagus and simmer for 5 minutes, before adding the spinach and mint. Cook for 1 minute until the spinach wilts into the broth. Check the seasoning, adding salt and pepper as needed.

4. Meanwhile, brush a griddle pan with the remaining olive oil and set over a medium heat. Add the salmon to the hot pan and cook for about 5 minutes on each side until the flesh is starting to flake and the skin is crisp and golden.

5. Divide the spring vegetable broth between 4 deep serving plates and top each one with the salmon. Serve immediately topped with a dollop of the herb mayonnaise.

OR YOU CAN TRY THIS...

- Instead of serving with the mayonnaise, stir pesto into the broth.

- Use chives or basil instead of mint, and sorrel rather than spinach.

SPINACH & SMOKED SALMON ROULADE

Cream cheese and ricotta contain moderate amounts of lactose, so if you malabsorb lactose you may wish to use half the quantity listed below and mix it with some mashed feta.

SERVES 4–6
PREP: 20 MIN
COOK: 25 MIN

butter, for greasing

400g/14oz spinach, trimmed

3 medium free-range eggs, separated

225g/8oz (1 cup) cream cheese or ricotta

110g/4oz smoked salmon, chopped

1 bunch of chives, chopped

grated zest of 1 lemon

FOR THE WHITE SAUCE:

4 tbsp cornflour (cornstarch)

600ml/1 pint (2½ cups) semi-skimmed milk or lactose-free milk

85g/3oz (scant ½ cup) virtually fat-free fromage frais

a pinch of ground nutmeg

salt and freshly ground black pepper

1. Preheat the oven to 190°C, 375°F, gas mark 5. Lightly grease a 20 x 30cm (8 x 12in) Swiss roll tin (jelly roll pan) with parchment paper (waxed paper).

2. Make the white sauce: blend the cornflour with a little of the milk to a smooth paste. Heat the remaining milk in a pan and as soon as it starts to boil, reduce the heat and stir in the cornflour mixture with a wooden spoon. Cook gently, stirring all the time, for about 3 minutes until the sauce is really smooth and thickens to a coating consistency. Remove from the heat and stir in the fromage frais and nutmeg. Season to taste and pour into a food processor.

3. Put the spinach leaves in a large saucepan with a spoonful of water and place over a medium heat. Cover the pan and cook for about 2 minutes, shaking the pan occasionally, until the leaves turn bright green and wilt. Drain in a colander, pressing down with a small plate to extract the excess moisture.

4. Add the spinach to the food processor and pulse briefly with the white sauce. Tip in the egg yolks and blitz until well blended. Transfer the mixture to a large mixing bowl.

⊙ ⊙ ⊙

SPINACH & SMOKED SALMON ROULADE

5. In a clean, dry bowl beat the egg whites until they form soft peaks. Fold gently but thoroughly into the spinach mixture in a figure-of-eight motion with a metal spoon. Tip into the prepared tin and cook in the preheated oven for about 15 minutes until the spinach roulade is well-risen and it springs back when lightly pressed with a finger. Set aside to cool.

6. Mix the cream cheese or ricotta with the smoked salmon, chives and lemon zest.

7. Invert the spinach roulade onto a large sheet of parchment paper (waxed paper) and peel away the backing paper. Spread the cheese and smoked salmon mixture over the roulade, not quite up to the edges.

8. Roll up the roulade, using the baking parchment to help you. Transfer to a serving plate, seam-side down, then cover and chill in the fridge for at least 2 hours before serving cut into slices.

OR YOU CAN TRY THIS...

- Mix the cooked spinach with some watercress or rocket (arugula) for a peppery flavour.

- Use smoked salmon trimmings – they are cheaper than slices.

- Instead of chives, use parsley, tarragon or basil.

- Serve with a fresh tomato coulis.

SMOKED HADDOCK FISH CAKES
WITH PARSLEY SAUCE

Homemade fish cakes are always popular – a little time-consuming to make perhaps, but well worth the effort. I usually make double the quantity, and freeze half for another meal. These fish cakes include bacon pieces and have a subtle smoky flavour. A parsley sauce is the traditional accompaniment.

SERVES 4
PREP: 20 MIN
COOK: 35–40 MIN

350g/12oz undyed smoked haddock

450g/1lb potatoes

6 rashers streaky bacon, derinded

30g/1oz (2 tbsp) butter

6 spring onions (scallions), green parts only, finely chopped

1 tbsp lemon juice

1 tbsp chopped fresh parsley

1 egg, beaten

60g/2oz (1 cup) fresh white gluten-free breadcrumbs

oil, for frying

salt and freshly ground black pepper

FOR THE PARSLEY SAUCE:
300ml/10½fl oz (1¼ cups) milk or lactose-free milk

1 bay leaf

6 peppercorns

1 tbsp cornflour (cornstarch)

60g/2oz (1⅓ cups) chopped fresh parsley

40g/1½oz (3 tbsp) butter

1. Place the haddock in a pan and add sufficient water to just cover. Bring to the boil, lower the heat and poach gently for 15–20 minutes, until the fish flakes.

2. Meanwhile, peel the potatoes, cut into even-sized pieces and cook in boiling salted water until tender. Drain well and mash until smooth.

3. Preheat the grill (broiler) and grill the bacon until just brown, but not crispy. Chop into small pieces.

4. Drain the fish and flake, discarding any bones and skin. Mix the fish with the mashed potatoes and bacon.

5. Melt the butter in a small pan, add the spring onion greens and cook until beginning to soften. Add to the fish mixture, with the lemon juice, parsley and seasoning. Add just enough beaten egg to bind the mixture; it must be firm enough to shape.

6. With floured hands, shape the mixture into 8 cakes. Brush with beaten egg and coat in the breadcrumbs. Chill in the refrigerator for 30 minutes.

7. To make the parsley sauce, put the milk in a pan with the bay leaf and peppercorns. Bring to the boil, turn off the heat, cover and leave to infuse for 10 minutes, then strain into a clean saucepan. Combine the cornflour with a couple of tablespoons water in a small bowl and mix until dissolved. Add it to the milk and bring to the boil, stirring until the sauce thickens. Stir in the chopped parsley, butter and seasoning to taste. Keep warm.

8. Heat the oil in a frying pan and shallow fry the fish cakes in batches if necessary, for about 5 minutes on each side, until golden and crisp. Drain on kitchen paper, then serve immediately, with the parsley sauce.

INDIAN MACKEREL
WITH SPICY POTATOES
& CARROT MASH

Mackerel is a great source of protein and omega-3, helping protect your heart and boosting your brain power. Don't be put off by the list of ingredients – it's a very easy dish to make and it doesn't take long.

SERVES 4
PREP: 15 MIN
MARINATE: 15 MIN
COOK: 20–25 MIN

juice of ½ lime

1 tbsp gluten-free curry paste

4 tbsp 0% fat Greek yoghurt or lactose-free yoghurt, plus extra to serve

4 large fresh mackerel fillets

1 tsp sunflower oil

1 small red chilli, deseeded and shredded

1 tsp cumin seeds

½ tsp black mustard seeds

½ tsp ground turmeric

salt and freshly ground black pepper

FOR THE SPICY POTATOES:
1 tbsp oil

500g/1lb 2oz potatoes, peeled and cubed

1 tsp ground turmeric

½ tsp chilli powder

FOR THE CARROT MASH:
500g/1lb 2oz carrots, sliced

½ tsp ground cumin

½ tsp ground turmeric

1 small bunch of coriander (cilantro), chopped

◉ ◉ ◉

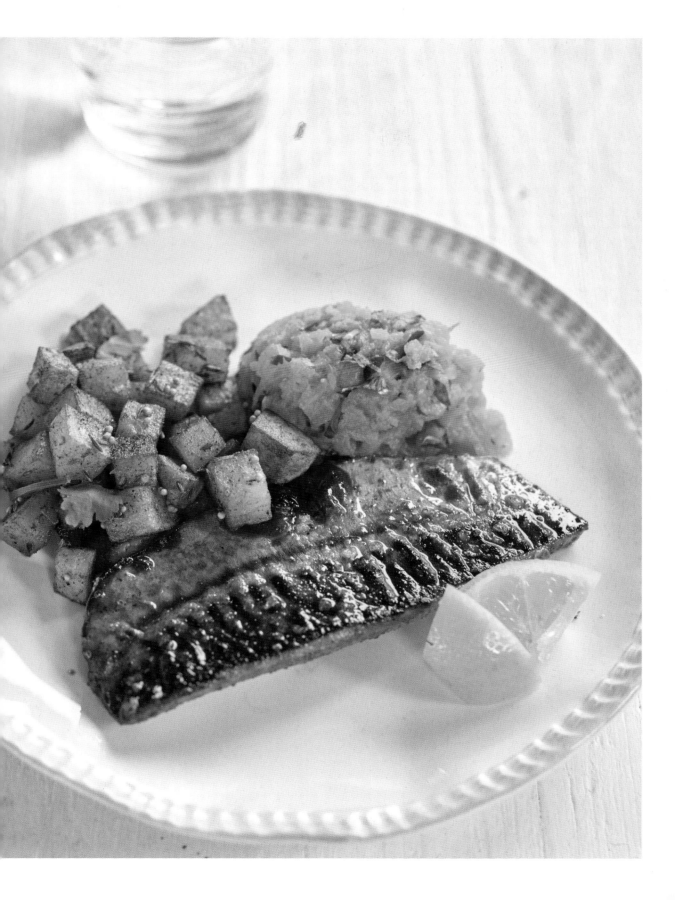

...INDIAN MACKEREL

1. Mix the lime juice, curry paste and yoghurt in a bowl. Add the mackerel and turn them in the marinade. Cover and leave in the fridge to marinate for at least 15 minutes.

2. Make the spicy potatoes: heat the oil in a large non-stick frying pan (skillet) over a medium to high heat and cook the potatoes for 5 minutes, stirring frequently, until golden brown. Stir in the turmeric and chilli powder and a good pinch of salt. Cover the pan and cook over a low heat for 10–15 minutes until the potatoes are tender.

3. Make the carrot mash: cook the carrots in lightly salted water for 10–15 minutes until tender. Drain well and mash with a fork or blitz in a blender. Stir in the spices and coriander.

4. Remove the mackerel fillets from the marinade and cook under a preheated hot grill (broiler) for 2–3 minutes each side until cooked.

5. Meanwhile, heat the oil in a frying pan (skillet) over a medium to high heat. Add the chilli and cook for 1 minute. Stir in the seeds and turmeric and cook for 1 minute until the mustard seeds start to pop and release their aroma.

6. Scatter over the mackerel and serve immediately with the carrot mash, spicy potatoes and a spoonful of yoghurt.

OR YOU CAN TRY THIS...

⊙ Use salmon fillets instead of mackerel.

⊙ Try serving this with a cucumber raita and Indian chutney or pickles.

⊙ Stir some snipped chives into the cooked potatoes.

GREEK ISLAND FISH STEW

In the Aegean, this fish stew is usually made with the catch of the day – whatever's available. The same goes for the vegetables and flavourings: lemons are often used instead of oranges, and herbs include rosemary, thyme, basil and oregano.

SERVES 6
PREP: 30 MIN
COOK: 50 MIN

1kg/2lb 4oz mixed fish, e.g. monkfish (anglerfish), cod, hake, grouper, sea bream, sea bass (striped bass), red or grey mullet or whiting, preferably left whole and scaled, cleaned and gutted

4 tbsp fruity olive oil, plus extra for drizzling

1 leek, green leaves only, shredded

2 large carrots, thickly sliced

2 celery stalks, diced

2 courgettes (zucchini), sliced

675g/1½lb potatoes, peeled and cut into chunks

450g/1lb ripe tomatoes, coarsely chopped

a pinch of crushed chilli (hot pepper) flakes

1.2 litres/40fl oz (5 cups) onion-free fish stock

a pinch of saffron threads

1 tbsp tomato paste (optional)

2 bay leaves

2 strips orange zest

juice of 1 orange

a handful of flat-leaf parsley, chopped

a handful of dill, chopped

salt and freshly ground black pepper

1. Wash the fish under the cold tap. Pat dry with kitchen paper (towels) and cut each one through the bone into several thick pieces.

2. Heat the oil in a large saucepan set over a low heat and cook the leek, carrots and celery for about 10 minutes, stirring occasionally, until softened but not browned. Stir in the courgettes, potatoes, tomatoes and chilli. Cook gently for 5 minutes and then add the stock, saffron, tomato paste (if using), bay leaves and orange zest.

3. Bring to the boil, then cover the pan and cook over a low heat for 15 minutes until the vegetables are tender. Add the fish and simmer for a further 10–15 minutes until the fish is thoroughly cooked, opaque and starting to come away from the bone. Add the orange juice and season to taste with salt and pepper.

4. Stir in the chopped herbs and ladle into shallow bowls, dividing the fish equally between them. Drizzle with a little olive oil and serve.

OR YOU CAN TRY THIS…

- Add some shellfish, too: mussels, clams, prawns (shrimp), meaty crab claws or even lobster if it's a special occasion.

- Enhance the flavour with a glass of red or white wine.

- A thinly sliced fennel bulb adds a subtle aniseed flavour.

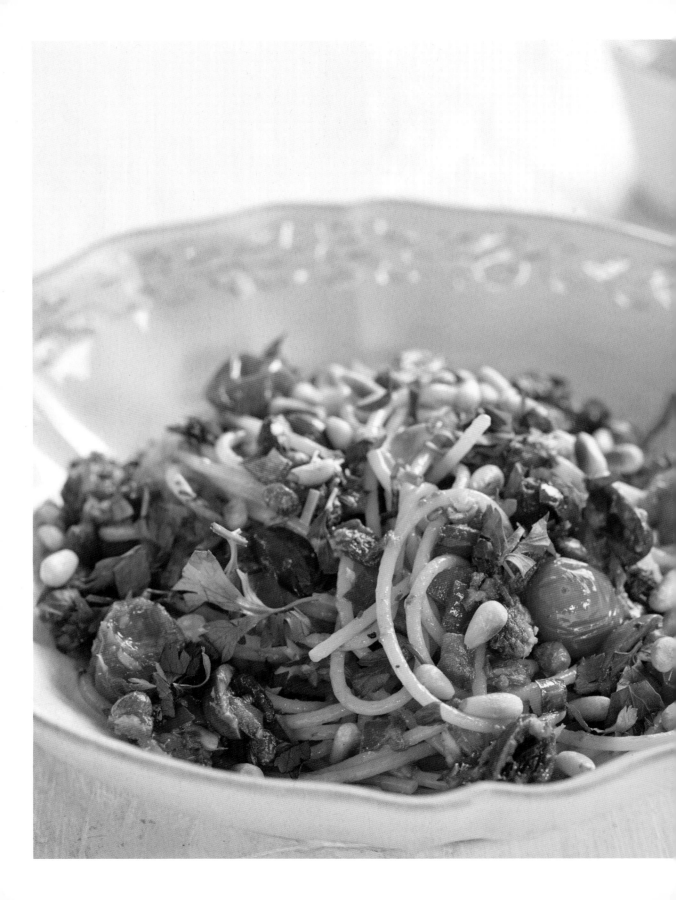

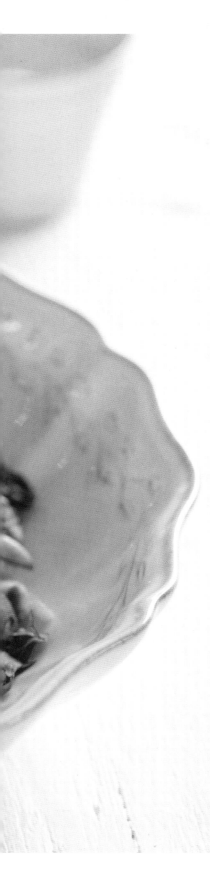

SICILIAN TOMATO & SARDINE SPAGHETTI

The *agrodolce* (sweet and sour) flavour is a feature of Sicilian cuisine. This quick weekday pasta dish is very economical to make and utilizes many basic store cupboard ingredients.

SERVES 4
PREP: 10 MIN
COOK: 18 MIN

2 tbsp olive oil

1 red (bell) pepper, deseeded and diced

1 tsp fennel seeds

a pinch of chilli (hot pepper) flakes

400g/14oz small plum tomatoes, quartered or halved

a pinch of sugar

1 tbsp red wine vinegar

2 x 110g/4oz cans boned sardines in olive oil, drained and cut in half

2 tbsp capers

12 black olives, stoned (pitted)

2 tbsp sultanas (golden raisins), soaked in hot water and drained

400g/14oz spaghetti (dry weight)

4 tbsp flat-leaf parsley, chopped

2 tbsp toasted pine nuts

salt and freshly ground black pepper

◦ ◦ ◦

··· SICILIAN TOMATO & SARDINE SPAGHETTI

1. Heat the olive oil in a deep frying pan (skillet) set over a medium heat and cook the red pepper with the fennel seeds and chilli flakes for 10 minutes until tender.

2. Stir in the tomatoes and sugar and cook for about 5 minutes until softened. Stir in the vinegar, sardines, capers, olives and sultanas and season with salt and pepper. Heat through for 2–3 minutes.

3. Meanwhile, cook the spaghetti in a pan of lightly salted boiling water according to the instructions on the packet. Drain well.

4. Gently toss the cooked spaghetti with the sardine and tomato sauce and sprinkle with parsley. Divide between 4 serving plates and scatter the toasted pine nuts over the top. Serve immediately.

OR YOU CAN TRY THIS...

- Use a diced or thinly sliced fennel bulb instead of red pepper.

- Add canned tomatoes instead of fresh.

- Use balsamic vinegar to add extra sweetness.

- Linguine, angel hair pasta, fettuccine or tagliatelle can be substituted for spaghetti.

- If wished, top with grated Parmesan, although the Italians seldom add cheese to fish dishes.

FISH PIE
WITH SAFFRON MASH

Here's another favourite with a difference. Chunks of cod, prawns and mussels are cooked in a creamy sauce under a layer of golden coloured saffron-scented mashed potato. The pie is flavoured with fresh dill and tomato, and is guaranteed to become a firm favourite!

SERVES 4–6
PREP: 25 MIN
COOK: 30–35 MIN

FOR THE SAFFRON MASH:

1kg/2¼lb floury potatoes

1 tsp saffron threads

75g/2½oz (5 tbsp) butter, melted

150ml/5fl oz (⅔ cup) single (light) cream

150ml/5fl oz (⅔ cup) milk

salt and freshly ground black pepper

FOR THE PIE FILLING:

450g/1lb cod fillet

480ml/16fl oz (2 cups) milk

1 bay leaf

225g/8oz tomatoes

180g/6oz cooked shelled prawns (shrimp)

180g/6oz cooked shelled mussels

1 tbsp chopped fresh dill

1½ tbsp cornflour (cornstarch)

50g/2oz (4 tbsp) butter

1. Preheat the oven to 180°C, 350°F, gas mark 4. For the saffron mash, peel the potatoes and cut into even-sized chunks. Put them in a pan with enough water to cover, and add the saffron. Bring to the boil and simmer, covered, until cooked.

2. Drain the potatoes, retaining the saffron. Add the butter and mash smoothly. Add the cream and milk and beat until light and fluffy. Season with salt and pepper to taste.

3. Meanwhile, lay the cod in an ovenproof dish, pour in the milk and add the bay leaf. Cover and cook in the oven for 20 minutes until the fish is firm. Strain off the milk and reserve.

4. In the meantime, plunge the tomatoes into boiling water for 30 seconds, then refresh in cold water and peel away the skins. Cut into quarters, remove the seeds and roughly chop the flesh.

5. Turn the oven up to 230°C, 450°F, gas mark 8. Flake the cod into a buttered ovenproof dish. Add the prawns, mussels and tomatoes. Scatter over the dill.

6. Put all but 2 tablespoons of the reserved poaching milk in a saucepan. Mix the 2 tablespoons of milk with the cornflour in a small bowl until the flour has dissolved. Stir the cornflour mixture into the reserved milk, and cook, stirring, until thickened. Add 3 tablespoons of the butter and let melt in, then season with salt and pepper. Pour the sauce over the fish.

7. Spoon the saffron mash on top of the fish mixture, covering it completely. Dot with the remaining butter and bake in the oven for 10–15 minutes until nicely browned on top.

NOTE: If using frozen prawns and mussels, defrost thoroughly in the fridge overnight; drain well before adding to the cod.

OR YOU CAN TRY THIS…

⊙ Omit the saffron. Flavour the mashed potato with some chopped fresh herbs, such as dill, tarragon and chervil.

CRISPY COD GOUJONS WITH TARTARE SAUCE

This healthy low FODMAP version of a universally popular dish uses gluten-free flour and breadcrumbs and grilled (broiled) – not deep-fried – fish goujons. You can use any firm-fleshed white fish, such as haddock or monkfish (anglerfish).

SERVES 4
PREP: 20 MIN
COOK: 10 MIN

600g/1lb 5oz thick cod fillets, skinned

gluten-free flour, for dusting, e.g. rice flour

4 egg whites

110g/4oz fresh gluten-free white breadcrumbs

spray oil

potatoes or rice, to serve

FOR THE TARTARE SAUCE:
2 free-range egg yolks

1 tsp Dijon mustard

a pinch of salt

120ml/4fl oz (½ cup) olive oil

120ml/4fl oz (½ cup) sunflower oil

2–3 tbsp lemon juice

3 tbsp chopped capers

4 small gherkins, finely chopped

a small bunch of chives, snipped

a few sprigs of dill, finely chopped

⊙ ⊙ ⊙

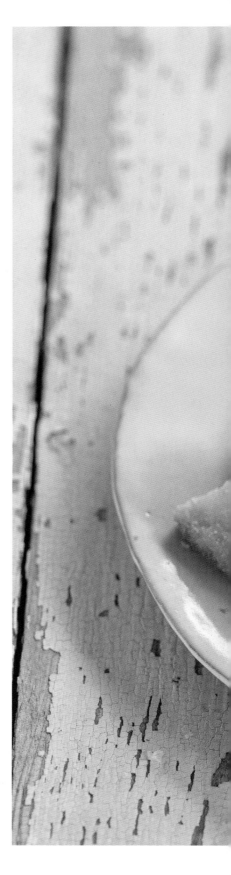

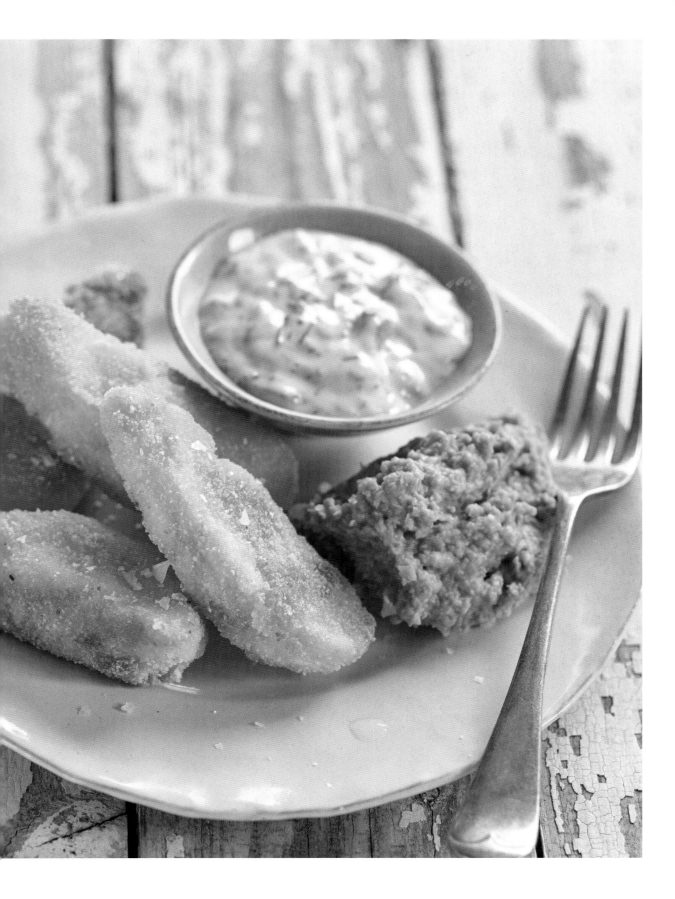

...CRISPY COD GOUJONS

1. Make the tartare sauce: in a food processor or blender, blitz the egg yolks, mustard and salt. On the slowest setting, add the oils gradually in a thin stream through the feed tube, beating all the time until you have a thick mayonnaise. Thin to the desired consistency with the lemon juice, then transfer to a bowl and stir in the remaining ingredients.

2. Check the cod fillets for any small bones and cut them into thick strips. Dust them lightly with flour.

3. In a clean, dry bowl, beat the egg whites until really stiff. Dip the cod strips into the beaten egg white. Spread the breadcrumbs out in a shallow dish and use to coat the cod, pressing them in gently all over.

4. Arrange the coated cod goujons on a foil-lined grill (broiler) pan and spray them lightly with oil.

5. Cook under a preheated hot grill (broiler) for 4–5 minutes each side, until golden brown and crisp and thoroughly cooked inside.

6. Serve the hot goujons with the tartare sauce and some potatoes or rice. A crisp salad or green vegetables makes a good accompaniment.

OR YOU CAN TRY THIS...

- Use cornichons or dill pickles instead of gherkins in the tartare sauce.

- The herbs you use in the sauce will dictate the flavour: try tarragon or parsley.

- Give the tartare sauce a kick with a dash of Tabasco or a pinch of cayenne.

STEAMED COD
WITH NOODLES

If you don't have a steamer, you can use a colander set over a saucepan of simmering water and cover it with a lid. Or wrap the fish and vegetables loosely in kitchen foil and place in simmering water to steam them. You will need thick fish fillets (not long thin ones) to make this dish.

SERVES 4
PREP: 10 MIN
COOK: 10 MIN

250g/9oz rice noodles (dry weight)

2 heads of pak choi (bok choy), halved or quartered

150g/5oz fine green beans, trimmed

4 thick cod fillets, skinned

3 tbsp light soy sauce

1 tbsp mirin

juice of ½ lime

1 tbsp sunflower oil

1 tsp caster (superfine) sugar

1 red chilli, deseeded and finely shredded

a few chives, to serve

1. Cook the noodles according to the instructions on the packet.

2. Meanwhile, arrange the pak choi and green beans on a heatproof plate and place it inside a steamer. Lay the cod fillets on top and steam for 10 minutes or until the vegetables are tender and the fish is thoroughly cooked and opaque.

3. Mix together the soy sauce, mirin, lime juice, oil, sugar and chilli in a small bowl to make a dressing.

4. Divide the vegetables and rice noodles between 4 serving plates and place the cod on top. Drizzle with the dressing and serve garnished with chives.

OR YOU CAN TRY THIS...

- Use haddock, sea bass or other white fish fillets.

- For a more intense flavour, swap the sunflower oil for sesame oil, or use a mixture of the two.

- You can use another rice wine vinegar or even balsamic instead of mirin.

- Snip the chives and add to the dressing.

- Use coriander (cilantro) or Thai basil instead of chives.

SPICY FISH FILLETS WITH SAAG ALOO

A spicy supper which isn't too hot – you can even leave out the chilli altogether if you prefer more subtle undertones of spice.

SERVES 4
PREP: 15 MIN
COOK: 20 MIN

1 tbsp coriander seeds

2 tsp black mustard seeds

1 tbsp fennel seeds

1 tsp ground turmeric

a pinch of ground ginger

4 thick white fish fillets, e.g. haddock or cod, skinned

sunflower oil, for brushing

salt and freshly ground black pepper

Greek yoghurt or lactose-free yoghurt, to serve

FOR THE SAAG ALOO:
2 tbsp sunflower oil

2.5cm/1in piece fresh root ginger, peeled and diced

1 red chilli, deseeded and shredded

1 tsp black mustard seeds

1 tsp cumin seeds

½ tsp fennel seeds

½ tsp ground turmeric

400g/14oz potatoes, peeled and cubed

300g/10½oz baby spinach leaves

◎ ◎ ◎

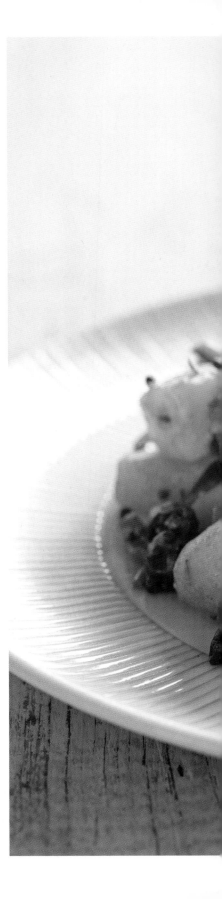

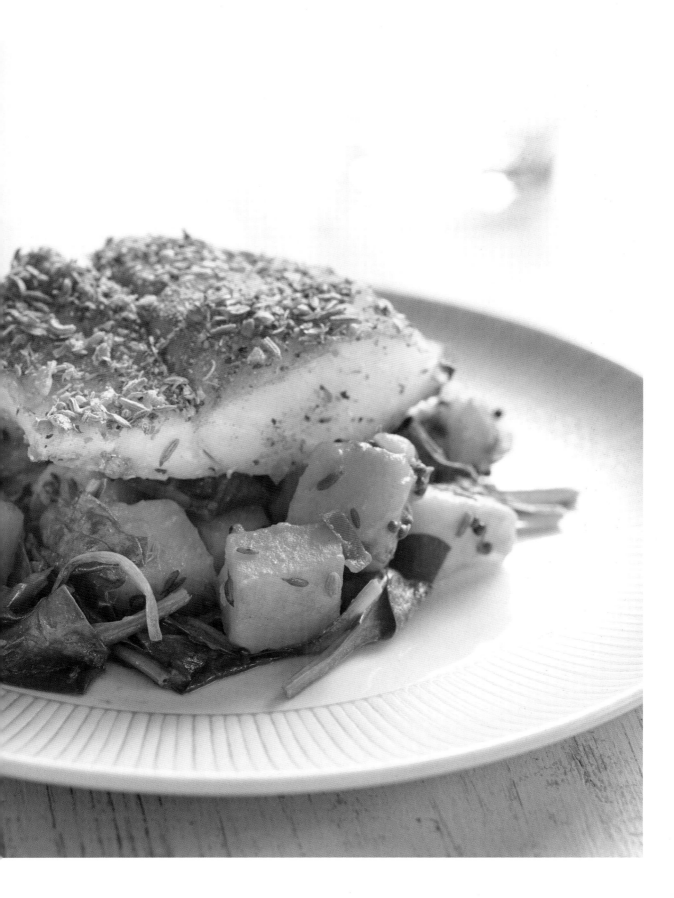

··· SPICY FISH FILLETS

1. Preheat the oven to 180°C, 350°F, gas mark 4.

2. Set a frying pan (skillet) over a medium heat and dry-fry the coriander and mustard seeds for 1 minute or until the mustard seeds begin to pop. Stir in the fennel seeds and heat for 30 seconds. Remove the seeds from the pan.

3. Grind the seeds coarsely in a pestle and mortar. Add the ground spices and grind until well mixed. Season with salt and pepper and sprinkle the over the fish fillets, lightly pressing the seeds into them all over.

4. Arrange the fish fillets on a lightly oiled baking (cookie) sheet. Bake in the preheated oven for 15–20 minutes, turning them once, until the fish is cooked through and the crust is crisp and golden.

5. Meanwhile, make the saag aloo. Heat the oil in a large frying pan (skillet) over a medium heat and cook the ginger and chilli for 2 minutes. Stir in the seeds, turmeric and potatoes and cook for 5 minutes, stirring occasionally. Add 2–3 tablespoons water, then cover the pan, reduce the heat and simmer for 8–10 minutes until the potatoes are tender. Stir in the spinach and as soon as it wilts and turns bright green remove from the heat.

6. Serve the spicy fish fillets and saag aloo and some cooling yoghurt.

OR YOU CAN TRY THIS...

- You can make this with skinned salmon or mackerel fillets.

- Add some chopped juicy tomatoes to the saag aloo.

JERKED PRAWNS WITH QUINOA

The nutty flavour and interesting texture of quinoa makes it a popular 'superfood'. High in protein and fibre, cholesterol- and gluten-free, it's the perfect way to create a filling FODMAP-friendly supper. You can serve this with a crisp salad or some steamed green beans.

SERVES 4
PREP: 20 MIN, PLUS CHILLING
COOK: 20 MIN

450g/1lb large raw shelled prawns (jumbo shrimp)

200g/7oz (scant 1¼ cups) quinoa (dry weight)

480ml/16fl oz (2 cups) onion-free fish or chicken stock

3 tbsp fruity olive oil

a small bunch of coriander (cilantro), chopped

1 small ripe avocado, peeled, stoned (pitted) and diced

juice of 1 lime

salt and freshly ground black pepper

FOR THE JERK SEASONING:

2 tsp allspice berries

2 tsp black peppercorns

a pinch of ground nutmeg

a pinch of ground cinnamon

leaves stripped from 4 sprigs of thyme

2.5cm/1in piece fresh root ginger, peeled and grated

1–2 chillies, diced, e.g. Scotch bonnet

2 tsp brown sugar

1 tbsp soy sauce

1 tsp garlic-infused olive oil

juice of 1 lime

1. Make the jerk seasoning: crush the allspice and peppercorns in a pestle and mortar, then place in a blender with the other ingredients and blitz to a paste.

2. Transfer to a bowl and add the prawns (shrimp), turning them until they are well coated. Cover and chill in the fridge for at least 30 minutes.

3. Meanwhile, rinse the quinoa under running cold water, then drain. Heat the stock in a saucepan and add the quinoa when it starts to boil. Reduce the heat, cover the pan and simmer gently for 15 minutes until tender and most of the liquid has been absorbed. Turn off the heat and leave to steam in the pan for 6–8 minutes before draining off any excess liquid. Fluff up the quinoa with a fork.

4. Add 2 tablespoons olive oil, the coriander, avocado and lime juice to the quinoa and mix gently together. Season to taste with salt and pepper.

5. Cook the prawns in their jerk marinade in the remaining oil in a large frying pan (skillet) over a medium to high heat or on a hot griddle or barbecue for 1–2 minutes each side until they are pink, juicy and succulent.

6. Spoon the quinoa onto 4 serving plates and arrange the prawns on top. Serve immediately.

OR YOU CAN TRY THIS...

- Serve the quinoa topped with griddled sliced chicken or lean, grilled (broiled) tuna or salmon marinated in soy sauce.

- Vegetarians can top the quinoa with griddled feta or tofu, or some roasted vegetables, e.g. peppers, squash, pumpkin, aubergines (eggplants) and courgettes (zucchini).

- Stir some chopped parsley, chives, dill or basil into the quinoa.

GRIDDLED SQUID
WITH SWEET POTATO WEDGES

If you are squeamish about cleaning the squid yourself, ask your fishmonger to do it for you or buy a packet of fresh or frozen ready-prepared squid.

SERVES 4
PREP: 15 MIN
COOK: 25–30 MIN

350g/12oz sweet potatoes, peeled and cut into wedges

75ml/2½fl oz (5 tbsp) olive oil

a few sprigs of rosemary

600g/1lb 5oz squid, cleaned

1 tsp black peppercorns, crushed, plus extra to season

1 tsp coarse sea salt flakes, crushed, plus extra to season

a pinch of dried chilli (hot pepper) flakes

85g/3oz wild rocket (arugula)

balsamic vinegar, for drizzling

1 lemon, cut into wedges

OR YOU CAN TRY THIS...

- Serve with roasted pumpkin or swede or even some aubergine (eggplant).

- Sprinkle the sweet potatoes with thyme.

- Use some sweet chilli sauce for dipping.

1. Preheat the oven to 200°C, 400°F, gas mark 6.

2. Arrange the sweet potatoes in a roasting tin (pan) and drizzle with 2 tablespoons of the olive oil. Tuck the rosemary down between the wedges and grind some sea salt and black pepper over the top. Bake in the preheated oven for 25–30 minutes until tender and golden brown.

3. Meanwhile, wash the squid under the running cold tap and pat dry with kitchen paper (towels). Cut off the tentacles and discard the hard 'beak' at their base. Cut off the 'ears' on either side of the 'hood' and peel away the skin. Slice open the hood and lay it out flat with the inner surface facing you. Score in a diamond pattern with a sharp knife.

4. Brush the squid pieces with olive oil and lightly press the crushed peppercorns, salt and chilli flakes into them.

5. Brush a griddle pan with the remaining oil and set over a high heat. When it's really hot, add the squid and cook for 1–2 minutes until just cooked and tender. Take care not to overcook it or it will become tough.

6. Serve immediately with the sweet potato wedges and the rocket drizzled with balsamic vinegar. Squeeze the lemon wedges over the hot squid.

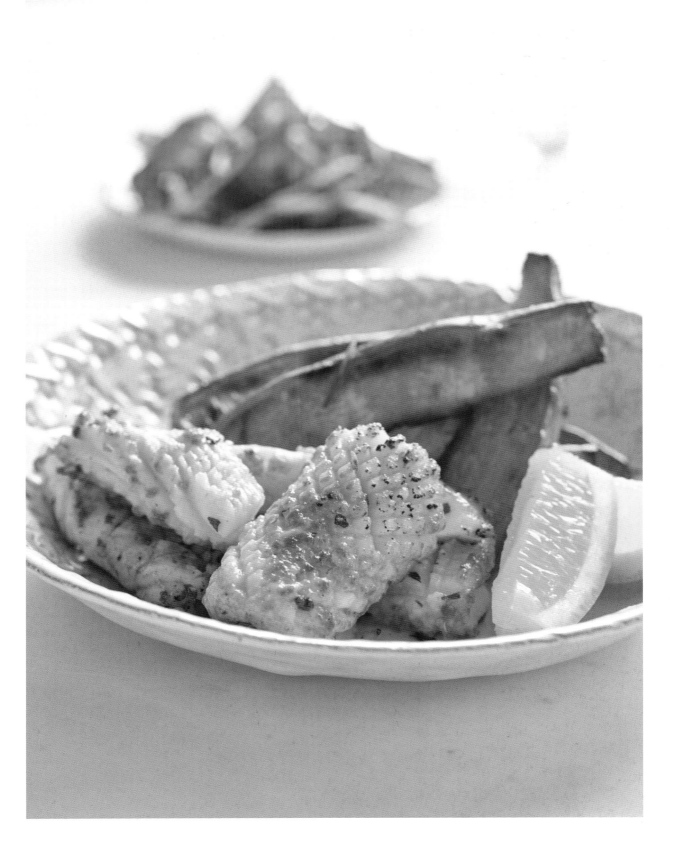

HERB RISOTTO WITH PRAWNS (SHRIMP)

For the best results, you must use a really good stock to make this risotto. Chicken or fish stock will do the trick if you don't have vegetable. Vegetarians can omit the prawns and serve the risotto topped with roasted or griddled FODMAP-friendly vegetables.

SERVES 4
PREP: 10 MIN
COOK: 35 MIN

a large bunch of mixed herbs, e.g. basil, chervil, chives, dill, flat-leaf parsley, tarragon

1.5 litres/52fl oz (6¼ cups) hot onion-free vegetable stock

2 tbsp olive oil

60g/2oz (3 tbsp) butter

1 small fennel bulb, diced

400g/14oz (scant 2 cups) risotto rice

a pinch of chilli powder

3½ tbsp white vermouth or wine

grated zest and juice of 1 lemon

4 tbsp crème fraîche or lactose-free crème fraîche

8 shelled large prawns (jumbo shrimp)

salt and freshly ground black pepper

grated Parmesan, to serve

1. Strip off the leaves off the stalks of the herbs. Chop the leaves and set aside. Make the stalks into a bundle and tie with string. Pour the vegetable stock into a large saucepan and add the herb-stalk bundle. Bring to the boil and then cover the pan and reduce the heat to a bare simmer.

2. Heat 1 tablespoon of the olive oil and the butter in a heavy-bottomed saucepan over a low heat. Add the fennel and cook gently, stirring occasionally, for about 10 minutes until softened.

3. Add the rice and chilli powder and stir until all the grains are glistening. Add the vermouth or wine and a ladleful of the hot stock and cook, stirring, over a low heat until the liquid is absorbed by the rice. Add another ladleful and keep stirring and adding more stock in this way until the rice is tender but *al dente* (it still has a little 'bite'). The risotto should have a moist consistency, but not be mushy.

4. Stir in most of the chopped herb leaves together with the lemon zest and juice. Season to taste with salt and pepper and stir in the crème fraîche.

5. Meanwhile, heat the remaining oil in a griddle pan or frying pan (skillet), add the prawns and cook for 1–2 minutes, turning halfway through, until they turn pink.

6. Divide the risotto between 4 deep serving plates. Top with the prawns and sprinkle with the remaining herbs and Parmesan.

OR YOU CAN TRY THIS…

- Add a pinch of saffron strands to the simmering herb stock and you'll have a golden risotto.

- Instead of prawns, top with slices of griddled chicken.

- Add some green vegetables for a really green risotto: diced or shredded courgettes (zucchini), fine green beans, rocket (arugula) or baby spinach.

LEMONY PRAWN & ROCKET SPAGHETTI

Serve this quick and stylish supper with a crisp salad. You can buy packs of frozen tiger prawns in the freezer aisle of the supermarket. Defrost them thoroughly before cooking.

SERVES 4
PREP: 5 MIN
COOK: 10 MIN

450g/1lb gluten-free spaghetti (dry weight)

1 tbsp olive oil

a good pinch of dried chilli (hot pepper) flakes

a handful of parsley, finely chopped

a small bunch of chives, snipped

grated zest and juice of 1 lemon

120ml/4fl oz (½ cup) dry white wine

2 tomatoes, diced

450g/1lb peeled raw tiger prawns (shrimp)

a handful of rocket (arugula)

salt and freshly ground black pepper

freshly grated Parmesan, to serve (optional)

1. Cook the pasta in a large pan of boiling salted water according to the instructions on the packet until just tender (*al dente*). Drain well.

2. Meanwhile, heat the oil in a large deep frying pan (skillet) over a medium heat. Add the chilli, chopped herbs, lemon juice, wine and tomatoes and bring to the boil. Let it bubble away and reduce for 3–4 minutes.

3. Add the prawns and rocket and cook for 2 minutes until the prawns turn pink and the rocket wilts. Season to taste with salt and pepper.

4. Toss with the drained spaghetti to coat all the strands and then ladle into shallow serving bowls. Serve immediately sprinkled with lemon zest and Parmesan (if using).

OR YOU CAN TRY THIS...

- Use any gluten-free pasta, such as linguine, tagliatelle or fettuccine.

- Baby spinach leaves can be substituted for the rocket.

- Use a tablespoon or two of tomato paste instead of diced tomatoes.

- Instead of prawns, add a defrosted pack of *fruits de mer* (prawns, mussels, scallops and squid).

COCONUT SHRIMP & TOMATO CURRY

This is a quick and delicious curry that you can easily make at home. If you don't have any prawns (shrimp), just add some leftover cooked chicken at the end.

SERVES 4
PREP: 15 MIN
COOK: 35–40 MINUTES

1 large aubergine (eggplant)

5 tbsp sunflower oil

2 red (bell) peppers, deseeded and diced

1 red chilli, diced

5cm/2in piece fresh root ginger, peeled and diced

1 tsp ground turmeric

½ tsp ground cinnamon

1 tsp garam masala

2 tsp crushed coriander seeds

1 tbsp black mustard seeds

450g/1lb ripe tomatoes, roughly chopped

400ml/14fl oz (1¾ cups) canned coconut milk

500g/1lb 2oz shelled large raw tiger prawns (jumbo shrimp)

225g/8oz baby leaf spinach

a handful of coriander (cilantro), roughly chopped

salt and freshly ground black pepper

boiled rice, to serve

1. Slice the aubergine and then cut each slice in half or into quarters. Drizzle with some of the oil and cook, a few pieces at a time, in a non-stick griddle pan, over a medium heat until golden brown on both sides. Remove and drain on kitchen paper (towels).

2. While the aubergine is cooking, heat the remaining oil in a deep frying pan (skillet), add the red peppers chilli and cook over a low to medium heat for 6–8 minutes until softened. Stir in the ginger, ground spices and coriander and mustard seeds, and cook for 2 minutes.

3. Stir in the tomatoes and coconut milk and simmer gently for 15 minutes until the liquid reduces and thickens. Add the aubergine, prawns and spinach and cook for 2–3 minutes until the prawns are uniformly pink and the spinach has wilted into the curry. Season to taste with salt and pepper.

4. Sprinkle with coriander and serve immediately with boiled rice.

OR YOU CAN TRY THIS...

- Use cubes of paneer or tofu instead of prawns.

- Make the curry more fiery by adding some hot curry paste.

- Use canned tomatoes instead of fresh ones.

- Add some sliced courgettes (zucchini) and cubed potatoes.

- You can eat this with some cooling lactose-free yoghurt or even stir in a couple of spoonfuls before serving.

- Spicy mango chutney goes well with this dish.

MOULES FRITES

There is nothing quite like sitting down to a bowl of plump mussels fried to a golden crunch in butter and breadcrumbs, and thin crisp *pommes frites*. Classic aioli may be off the cards for a FODMAP diet, but if you make your own mayonnaise using garlic-infused oil, you can go some way to replicating that traditional accompaniment.

SERVES 4–6
PREP: 45 MIN, PLUS SOAKING
COOK: ABOUT 30 MIN

2.3kg/5lb mussels in shells, or 900g/2lb cooked shelled mussels

3 egg yolks

1 egg white

180–225g/6–8oz fresh white gluten-free breadcrumbs

900g/2lb potatoes, such as Désirée, King Edward or Maris Piper

oil, for deep-frying

225g/8oz (scant 1 cup) butter

salt and freshly ground black pepper

lemon wedges, to serve

FOR THE MAYONNAISE
2 egg yolks

210ml/7fl oz (¾ cup) garlic-infused oil

210ml/7fl oz (¾ cup) sunflower oil

squeeze of lemon juice, to taste

◦ ◦ ◦

⚬⚬⚬ MOULES FRITES

1. Clean the mussels thoroughly under cold running water and pull away any 'beards'. Soak in a bowl, of cold water for at least 30 minutes.

2. Meanwhile, make the mayonnaise. Put the egg yolks in a blender or food processor with a pinch of salt and blend until smooth. With the motor running, pour in half of the oil in a thin steady stream until the mixture starts to thicken. Add lemon juice and add the rest of the oil more boldly until it is all incorporated and the mayonnaise is thick. Check the seasoning. Set aside in a cool place, not the refrigerator.

3. After soaking, drain the mussels and tap each opened one sharply with the back of a knife; discard any that do not close. Place the mussels in a large saucepan with 300ml/10½fl oz (1¼ cups) water. Cover tightly and cook over a high heat, shaking the pan frequently for 5–8 minutes until the mussels open; do not overcook. Drain, discarding any unopened ones. Remove the mussels from their shells and pat dry.

4. Beat the egg yolks and white together in a bowl with a little salt, then add the mussels and toss to coat. Spread the breadcrumbs out on a tray and roll the mussels in them to coat evenly. Chill in the refrigerator.

5. Peel the potatoes and cut into 5mm/¼in slices. Stack 3–4 slices on top of each other, cut into thin chips, then immerse in a bowl of cold water. Repeat with the remaining potatoes. Rinse well, drain and pat very dry.

6. Half-fill a deep-fat fryer (with chip basket) with oil and heat to 150°C/300°F. Fry the potatoes in small batches for 4–7 minutes depending on thickness, until tender, but not coloured. Lift out and drain.

7. Melt half the butter in a large frying pan. When foaming, quickly fry half the mussels until golden brown, transfer to a warmed plate, while frying the rest.

8. Meanwhile, raise the temperature of the oil to 185°C/360°F and fry the potatoes for a further 30 seconds–2 minutes until golden brown and crisp. Drain on kitchen paper (towels) and sprinkle with salt. Serve immediately, with the mussels, mayonnaise and lemon wedges.

SEAFOOD RISOTTO

For the best flavour you should use the freshest fish and shellfish you can find. All shellfish are permissible on the FODMAP diet and they are a good source of zinc and selenium, which keep your immune system healthy. You can even add a defrosted packet of frozen *fruits de mer* if you're in a hurry.

SERVES 4
PREP: 25 MIN
COOK: 50 MIN

1kg/2lb 4oz fresh mussels in their shells

30g/1oz (2 tbsp) butter, plus extra for finishing

2 tbsp olive oil or garlic-infused oil

1 small fennel bulb, trimmed and thinly sliced

2 celery stalks, diced

450g/1lb fresh or frozen and thawed squid,
    cut into pieces

a pinch of chilli (hot pepper) flakes

225g/8oz (1 cup) arborio or carnaroli risotto rice
    (dry weight)

120ml/4fl oz (½ cup) dry white wine or vermouth,
    e.g. Noilly Prat

960ml/32fl oz (4 cups) hot simmering onion-free
    fish stock

a pinch of saffron threads

225g/8oz baby plum tomatoes, halved

350g/12oz large raw prawns (jumbo shrimp)

juice of 1 lemon

a small bunch of parsley, chopped

salt and freshly ground black pepper

◎ ◎ ◎

1. Scrub the mussels in a bowl of cold water, discarding any that are cracked or open. Place in a large saucepan with a little water. Bring to the boil, then cover the pan and cook for 4–5 minutes, shaking the pan occasionally, until they open – throw away any that stay closed. Remove about half the mussels from their shells and set aside, together with the remaining ones in their shells.

2. Heat the butter and oil in a heavy-bottomed large, deep frying pan (skillet) and cook the fennel and celery over a low heat, stirring occasionally, for 5 minutes until tender but not coloured.

3. Add the squid and cook gently for about 8 minutes, stirring occasionally, until tender. Stir in the chilli and rice and cook for 2–3 minutes until the grains start to crackle. Pour in the wine or vermouth and increase the heat. Cook rapidly for 2–3 minutes until the liquid reduces and evaporates.

4. Reduce the heat to a bare simmer and add a ladleful of the hot simmering stock with the saffron. Cook gently, stirring, until all the liquid has been absorbed. Add another ladle of stock and continue stirring and adding more stock until the rice is tender but not too soft – it should still have a little 'bite'.

5. Stir in the tomatoes, prawns and reserved mussels. Cook for 2–3 minutes until the prawns turn uniformly pink and the tomatoes start to soften.

6. Remove the pan from the heat and season to taste with salt and pepper. Stir in the lemon juice, parsley and a knob of butter. Cover the pan and set aside for 5 minutes before serving.

OR YOU CAN TRY THIS...

- Use fresh clams instead of mussels or even bottled clams if you can't get fresh ones.

- Add a cooked dressed crab, some scallops or chunks of white fish, red mullet or whole langoustines.

- If you like tomato-flavoured risotto, add 2 tablespoons tomato paste with the first ladle of stock.

KEDGEREE WITH HERB BUTTER

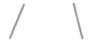

This simple combination of basmati rice, lightly poached smoked haddock, boiled eggs and subtle spice makes a lovely combination that's perfect for a light lunch, or more traditionally a breakfast dish to set you up for the day! The cockles and lemony herb butter provide additional flavour. As a more substantial main course this recipe will serve 2–3.

SERVES 4
PREP: 10 MIN
COOK: 20 MIN

450g/1lb smoked haddock (see note)

150ml/5fl oz (⅔ cup) milk

85g/3oz cooked cockles or clams

1 tsp coriander seeds

3 hard-boiled eggs

225g/8oz (1 cup) basmati rice (dry weight)

2 tbsp double (heavy) cream

3–4 tbsp chopped fresh chives, plus extra to garnish

salt and freshly ground black pepper

lemon or lime wedges, to garnish

FOR THE HERB BUTTER:
60g/2oz (4 tbsp) butter

1–2 tsp lemon juice

2 tbsp chopped fresh tarragon

1. Place the smoked haddock in a shallow pan with the milk. Cover and simmer gently for about 8 minutes until cooked through. Drain, reserving 2–3 tablespoons of the juices. Roughly flake the fish, discarding the skin and any bones.

2. Thoroughly drain the cockles. Finely crush the coriander seeds. Shell and quarter the eggs.

3. Cook the rice in plenty of boiling, salted water for 10 minutes or until just tender. Drain, rinse with boiling water and drain well.

4. Return the rice to the pan and add the flaked haddock, reserved cooking juices, cockles, coriander seeds, quartered eggs, cream and chives. Season lightly with salt and pepper and heat through gently for 2 minutes.

5. Meanwhile, for the herb butter, melt the butter and stir in the lemon juice, tarragon and a little seasoning. Pour into a warmed jug.

6. Spoon the kedgeree onto warmed serving plates and garnish with lemon or lime wedges and extra herbs. Serve accompanied by the herb butter.

OR YOU CAN TRY THIS...
- Use fresh salmon instead of smoked haddock.

- Replace the tarragon in the herb butter with dill or chervil.

NOTE: Choose natural undyed smoked haddock where possible. It's very pale by comparison to the familiar yellow smoked haddock, because it doesn't contain colouring and it generally has a superior flavour.

SUPPERS
=
VEGETABLES

THAI GREEN HOTPOT WITH RICE NOODLES

All you need to make this healthy supper are really fresh vegetables, some good-quality vegetable stock, flavourings and a pack of rice noodles. A fresh-tasting, zingy broth, it will detox and energize you on a cold day.

SERVES 4
PREP: 10 MIN
COOK: 20 MIN

2 pak choi (bok choy)

225g/8oz rice noodles (dry weight)

3 tbsp groundnut (peanut) oil or garlic-infused oil

1 large aubergine (eggplant), cut into cubes

2.5cm/1in piece fresh root ginger, peeled and diced

1 lemongrass stalk, peeled and finely sliced

1 red chilli, shredded

480ml/16fl oz (2 cups) hot onion-free vegetable stock

juice of 1 lime

2 tbsp nam pla (Thai fish sauce)

1 tbsp light soy sauce

a pinch of sugar

110g/4oz mangetout (snow peas), trimmed

110g/4oz baby spinach leaves

110g/4oz (1 cup) beansprouts

a handful of coriander (cilantro), chopped

1. Cut each pak choi (bok choy) into 4 wedges lengthwise. Cook in a pan of boiling salted water for 2–3 minutes until just tender but still slightly crisp. Plunge into a bowl of cold water, then drain well and set aside.

2. Put the rice noodles in a bowl and pour boiling water over them. Set aside for at least 10 minutes or follow the instructions on the packet.

3. Meanwhile, heat the oil in a large saucepan and cook the aubergine (eggplant) over a medium heat for 5 minutes, stirring occasionally, until just tender and golden brown.

4. Add the ginger, lemongrass and chilli to the pan and cook, stirring, for 2–3 minutes without colouring. Pour in the hot broth, lime juice, nam pla and soy sauce and simmer for 5 minutes. Add the mangetout and cook gently for 3–4 minutes until just tender.

5. Stir in the rice noodles, spinach, beansprouts and pak choi and cook for 2 minutes – just long enough for the spinach to wilt and to heat the noodles and vegetables.

6. Stir in the coriander and ladle into 4 shallow bowls.

OR YOU CAN TRY THIS...

- Make it more filling by adding griddled tofu, cooked chicken or prawns (shrimp).

- Don't add the noodles – serve the hotpot on a mound of rice.

- Give it a Japanese twist with mirin, teriyaki or tamari sauce.

- Make it spicy with a spoonful of Thai green curry paste.

- Add some courgette (zucchini) or Chinese leaves (Chinese cabbage).

PUMPKIN & SPINACH LASAGNE

You can assemble this delicious vegetarian lasagne in advance, then cover and keep in the fridge until you're ready to cook it. The flourless and fatless white sauce is made with FODMAP-friendly cornflour (cornstarch), making it healthier with less calories than usual.

SERVES 4
PREP: 15 MIN
COOK: 45–50 MIN

2 tbsp olive oil

1kg/2lb 4oz pumpkin, peeled, deseeded and
 cut into chunks

2 x 400g/14oz cans chopped tomatoes

2 tbsp tomato paste

a handful of parsley, chopped

a few drops of balsamic vinegar

250g/9oz spinach, trimmed and washed

12 sheets gluten-free lasagne (dried)

butter, for greasing

4 tbsp grated Parmesan cheese

salt and freshly ground black pepper

FOR THE WHITE SAUCE:
4 tbsp cornflour (cornstarch)

600ml/1 pint (2 ½ cups) skimmed milk or
 lactose-free milk

100g/3½oz (scant ½ cup) virtually fat-free
 fromage frais or lactose-free plain yoghurt

a pinch of ground nutmeg

○ ○ ○

PUMPKIN & SPINACH LASAGNE

1. Preheat the oven to 180°C, 350°F, gas mark 4.

2. Heat the oil in a large frying pan (skillet) over a low heat , add the pumpkin and cook, stirring occasionally, for 8–10 minutes until softened. Add the tomatoes, tomato paste and parsley and simmer gently for 10 minutes until the pumpkin is tender and the sauce thickens. Add a little balsamic vinegar and season with salt and pepper.

3. Cook the spinach with 1 tablespoon water in a covered saucepan over a medium heat, shaking the pan occasionally, for 2–3 minutes until the leaves wilt and turn bright green. Drain well in a colander, pressing down with a saucer to extract any excess water.

4. Meanwhile, make the white sauce: blend the cornflour with a little of the milk to a smooth paste. Heat the remaining milk in a pan and when it starts to boil, reduce the heat and stir in the cornflour mixture. Cook gently, stirring with a wooden spoon, for 2–3 minutes until the sauce is thick and smooth. Off the heat, stir in the fromage frais, nutmeg and seasoning.

5. Place 4 lasagne sheets in the bottom of a buttered large baking dish and pour half the pumpkin and tomato mixture over the top. Add half the spinach and then another layer of lasagne and spread with half the white sauce. Cover with the remaining pumpkin and tomato mixture and then the rest of the spinach and lasagna. Spoon the remaining white sauce over the top and sprinkle with Parmesan.

6. Bake in the preheated oven for 25–30 minutes until piping hot and golden brown. Serve cut into slices.

OR YOU CAN TRY THIS...

- Use fresh tomatoes instead of canned, with basil rather than parsley.

- Sprinkle the lasagne with grated Cheddar cheese.

TERIYAKI VEGETABLES WITH SESAME RICE NOODLES

Broccoli is allowed in small quantities on the low FODMAP diet. It's a moderate-fructan food and you can eat up to 100g/3½oz per portion.

SERVES 4
PREP: 10 MIN
COOK: 10 MIN

250g/9oz rice noodles (dry weight)

2 tbsp sesame oil

250g/9oz tenderstem broccoli or broccoli florets

200g/7oz fine green beans, trimmed

200g/7oz baby carrots, halved or quartered

1 tbsp toasted sesame seeds

FOR THE TERIYAKI SAUCE:

3 tbsp soy sauce

1 tbsp mirin

½ tsp sugar

2.5cm/1in piece fresh root ginger, peeled and diced

1. Cook the rice noodles according to the instructions on the packet.

2. Make the teriyaki sauce: mix all the ingredients together in a small bowl, stirring until blended.

3. Heat the sesame oil in a wok or frying pan (skillet) over a medium to high heat and stir-fry the broccoli, beans and carrots for 4–5 minutes until just tender. Stir in the teriyaki sauce and stir-fry for 1–2 minutes.

4. Add the cooked rice noodles and toss everything gently together until the noodles are lightly coated with the sauce.

5. Ladle into 4 serving bowls and serve sprinkled with sesame seeds.

OR YOU CAN TRY THIS...

- Use garlic-infused oil to stir-fry the vegetables.

- Add protein with some prawns (shrimp), chicken or tofu.

- Add thinly sliced (bell) peppers or courgette (zucchini).

SQUASH & TOMATO PENNE

Pasta always makes a tasty simple supper with minimal preparation. The gluten-free sort, which is usually made with rice, tastes just as good and is less bloating than traditional durum wheat pasta.

SERVES 4
PREP: 10 MIN
COOK: 20 MIN

2 tbsp olive oil

1 red (bell) pepper, deseeded and diced

600g/1lb 5oz butternut squash, peeled, deseeded and cubed

1 x 400g/14oz can chopped tomatoes

1 tbsp tomato paste

a good pinch of sugar

a few sprigs of parsley, chopped

60g/2oz lean bacon lardons (pieces)

350g/12oz gluten-free penne or pasta tubes (dry weight)

salt and freshly ground black pepper

Parmesan cheese shavings, to serve

1. Heat the olive oil in a large frying pan (skillet) over a low to medium heat and cook the red pepper and butternut squash, stirring occasionally, for 5 minutes until slightly softened.

2. Add the tomatoes and tomato paste with a pinch of sugar and cook for 8–10 minutes until the sauce has reduced and the squash is tender. Season with salt and pepper and stir in the chopped parsley.

3. In a small pan, dry-fry the bacon lardons – they will cook in their own fat. When they are crisp and golden, remove and drain on kitchen paper (towels) and keep warm.

4. Meanwhile, cook the pasta according to the instructions on the packet. Drain well and stir into the tomato and squash mixture. Fold in the bacon.

5. Divide between 4 serving plates and shave the Parmesan cheese over the top.

OR YOU CAN TRY THIS...

- Flavour the tomato sauce with a pinch of chilli (hot pepper) flakes or a drizzle of balsamic vinegar.

- Toss the sauce with some gluten-free spaghetti or linguine.

- Use chopped basil, oregano or sage instead of parsley.

- Make it more aromatic with garlic-infused olive oil.

- Use fresh tomatoes instead of canned.

CHEAT'S VEGGIE PASTA STACKS

Serve these quickly cooked and assembled stacks with some tomato sauce. If you don't want to make it yourself or don't have any in the freezer, you can heat up some passata and enhance it with some chopped basil and a dash of balsamic vinegar.

SERVES 4
PREP: 15 MIN
COOK: 10 MIN

16 sheets gluten-free lasagne (dried)

500g/1lb 2oz spinach, trimmed and washed

180g/6oz (¾ cup) ricotta cheese

180g/6oz feta cheese, mashed

a good pinch of grated nutmeg

grated zest of 1 lemon

a small bunch of chives, snipped

300g/10½oz fine green beans, trimmed

2 large courgettes (zucchini), cut into long matchsticks

8 asparagus spears, halved

salt and freshly ground black pepper

tomato sauce, to serve

1. Cook the lasagne in a large pan of boiling water for 7–10 minutes until just tender but not soft. It should be *al dente* (still have a little 'bite'). Remove with a slotted spoon and drain well.

2. While the pasta is cooking, put the spinach leaves in a large saucepan with a spoonful of water and place over a medium heat. Cover the pan and cook for about 2 minutes, shaking the pan occasionally, until the leaves turn bright green and wilt. Drain in a colander, pressing down with a small plate to extract the excess moisture.

3. Chop the spinach and mix with the ricotta, feta, nutmeg, lemon zest and chives. Season with salt and pepper.

4. Steam the green beans, courgettes and asparagus for a few minutes until just tender.

5. Assemble the lasagne stacks: place one sheet of lasagne on each serving plate and spread with a spoonful of the spinach mixture and some beans and courgettes. Cover with another sheet of lasagna and keep layering up in this way, topping each stack with a little spinach mixture and the asparagus.

6. Serve immediately with some tomato sauce.

OR YOU CAN TRY THIS…

- Use baby carrots, peppers or chunks of cooked pumpkin, squash or swede.

- Sprinkle the stacks with grated Parmesan.

- If you're watching your figure, you can mix the spinach with cottage cheese.

SOY-ROASTED CARROTS WITH TZATZIKI

Pouches of ready-to-eat rice and grains, which only need heating in a microwave, are perfect for a quick and easy supper. They come in many varieties and flavours, but check the ingredients on the label to make sure they don't include wheat, spelt, couscous, freekeh or barley.

SERVES 4
PREP: 15 MIN
COOK: 20 MIN

675g/1½lb small carrots, e.g. Chantenay

1 tbsp olive oil

1 tbsp soy sauce

1 tbsp maple syrup

2 tsp ground cumin

2 x 250g/9oz pouches ready-to-eat grains, e.g. wholegrain rice, quinoa, red rice and quinoa

salt and freshly ground black pepper

FOR THE TZATZIKI:
200g/7oz (1 cup) 0% fat Greek yoghurt or lactose-free low-fat yoghurt

½ cucumber, halved, deseeded and diced

1 tbsp garlic-infused olive oil

a handful of dill, chopped

a handful of parsley, chopped

1. Preheat the oven to 200°C, 400°F, gas mark 6.

2. Peel the carrots and trim the tops and tips. Cut each carrot in half lengthways.

3. Mix together the olive oil, soy sauce, maple syrup and cumin and use to coat the carrots. Arrange them in a roasting tin (pan) or ovenproof dish and cook in the preheated oven for about 20 minutes until tender and glossy, turning them halfway through cooking.

4. Meanwhile, make the tzatziki: mix all the ingredients together in a bowl and season to taste with salt and pepper.

5. Heat the grains in a microwave according to the instructions on the packet and divide between 4 shallow bowls. Arrange the carrots on top and serve with the tzatziki.

OR YOU CAN TRY THIS…

- You could roast some parsnips, sweet potatoes, squash or cauliflower florets in the same way.

- Serve the carrots on boiled nutty brown rice, quinoa or polenta cooked in the usual way.

SPINACH, STILTON & WALNUT PASTA

This tasty main course can be prepared and cooked in a matter of minutes. Blue cheeses, such as Stilton, are generally safe for those who are sensitive to lactose as the long ageing process means the lactose is hugely depleted. Serve as soon as it is ready, accompanied by a mixed salad.

SERVES 4
PREP: 10 MIN
COOK: 12 MIN

350g/12oz gluten-free pasta (dry weight)

250g/9oz spinach, stalks removed

250g/9oz ricotta cheese

a splash of milk

2 tbsp chopped thyme leaves

½ tsp ground allspice

120g/4½oz Stilton cheese, crumbled

60g/2oz walnuts, roughly chopped

coarse sea salt and freshly ground black pepper

1. Cook the pasta in a large pan of boiling salted water, according to the packet instructions until *al dente*, tender but still firm to the bite.

2. While the pasta is cooking, put the spinach in a steamer and steam for a couple of minutes until just wilted.

3. Put the ricotta in a pan and add a splash of milk to loosen it. Add the thyme and allspice and season really well with black pepper and a little salt (remembering that the Stilton is quite salty). Heat gently to warm.

4. Put the walnuts in a small dry frying pan and toast over a medium heat for a few minutes until they begin to smell toasty.

5. Drain the pasta thoroughly in a colander, then return to the hot pan. Pour over the ricotta mixture and stir in the wilted spinach. Add the crumbled Stilton and stir through just before serving, sprinkled with the toasted walnuts.

OR YOU CAN TRY THIS...

- For a more peppery flavour, switch the spinach for rocket (arugula) leaves and just let them wilt into the hot pasta.

- Use hazelnuts or pecans instead of the walnuts.

- Replace the Stilton with crumbled soft goat's cheese.

TOFU STIR-FRY
IN CHILLI SAUCE

Versatile and delicately flavoured, tofu is made from soy bean curd and is sold in white blocks. A good source of vegetable protein, it's high in iron and other minerals. You can marinate it before stir-frying or grilling (broiling), or add it to clear aromatic soup, stews and curries.

SERVES 4
PREP: 15 MIN, PLUS
MARINATING
COOK: 6–8 MIN

350g/12oz firm tofu, cubed

1 chilli, deseeded and chopped

75ml/2½fl oz (5 tbsp) groundnut (peanut) or sunflower oil

300g/10½oz rice noodles (dry weight)

1 tsp grated fresh root ginger

1 carrot, cut into thin matchsticks

32 mangetout (snow peas), trimmed and halved (8 pods each)

½ head broccoli, cut into florets

400g/14oz small pak choi (bok choy), quartered

2 tbsp light soy sauce

1 tbsp sweet chilli sauce

2 tbsp sesame seeds, to serve

1. Put the tofu in a bowl with the chilli and oil and stir until well coated. Leave to marinate for 20–30 minutes.

2. Cook the rice noodles according to the instructions on the packet.

3. Drain the marinade into a hot wok or frying pan (skillet) set over a medium to high heat. Add the ginger, carrot, mangetout, broccoli and pak choi and stir-fry for 3–4 minutes until slightly tender but still crisp. Add the soy sauce and sweet chilli sauce. Stir in the cooked rice noodles. Divide the mixture between 4 serving bowls.

4. Add the tofu to the wok and stir-fry for 2–3 minutes until golden and crisp all over. Spoon over the noodles and vegetables and serve sprinkled with sesame seeds.

OR YOU CAN TRY THIS...

- Serve with boiled or steamed rice instead of noodles.

- For a more delicate flavour, omit the sweet chilli sauce or pass it round for people to drizzle.

- Add a thinly sliced red, green or yellow (bell) pepper.

CHEESY SQUASH & TOMATO BAKE

This vegetarian gratin can be assembled a couple of hours in advance, ready to bake in the oven for the final 15 minutes just before serving supper. The best goat's cheese to use for this is a log of chèvre – it's easy to slice and turns appetizingly soft and golden brown when baked.

SERVES 4
PREP: 15 MIN
COOK: 40–45 MIN

900g/2lb butternut squash, peeled, deseeded and cubed

2 tsp fresh thyme leaves

2 tsp cumin seeds

240ml/8fl oz (1 cup) onion-free vegetable stock

120ml/4fl oz (½ cup) half-fat crème fraîche

85g/3oz soft goat's cheese

4 tbsp fresh gluten-free breadcrumbs

FOR THE TOMATO SAUCE:

2 tbsp olive oil

2 celery stalks, diced

1 red (bell) pepper, deseeded and finely diced

450g/1lb (2 cups) canned chopped tomatoes

1 tbsp tomato paste

1 tsp sugar

a few sprigs of basil, chopped

a drizzle of good balsamic vinegar

salt and freshly ground black pepper

1. Preheat the oven to 180°C, 350°F, gas mark 4.

2. Put the butternut squash in a large ovenproof dish and sprinkle with the thyme and cumin seeds. Season lightly with salt and black pepper and pour the stock over the top. Bake in the preheated oven for 25–30 minutes until just tender but not soft. Remove and turn up the oven to 200°C, 400°F, gas mark 6.

3. Meanwhile, make the tomato sauce. Heat the oil in a large frying pan (skillet) , add the celery and red pepper and cook over a low heat, stirring occasionally, for 8–10 minutes until softened. Stir in the tomatoes, tomato paste and sugar and simmer gently for 10 minutes until the sauce reduces and thickens. Add the basil and a glug of balsamic vinegar and season to taste with salt and pepper.

4. Pour the tomato sauce over the squash. Add small spoonfuls of crème fraîche and goat's cheese on top and sprinkle with the breadcrumbs.

5. Bake in the preheated oven for 15 minutes until the cheese melts, the breadcrumbs are crisp and golden and the sauce is bubbling. Serve hot or lukewarm with a crisp salad.

OR YOU CAN TRY THIS…

- Use swede, pumpkin or parsnips instead of butternut squash.

- Top with diced or sliced buffalo mozzarella instead of goat's cheese.

- Make the sauce with fresh ripe tomatoes instead of canned ones.

BUTTERNUT SQUASH RISOTTO

Make this comforting and unctuous dish in autumn when squash is in season and plentiful. Pumpkin is equally good and, if using, you can double the quantity to 400g/14oz, or use a mixture of half pumpkin (200g/7oz) and half squash (200g/7oz). The most important things to remember are not to rush and to use the best and freshest ingredients: good-quality stock and balsamic vinegar, risotto rice, freshly grated Parmesan. This is Italian slow food at its best.

SERVES 4
PREP: 10 MIN
COOK: 35–40 MIN

200g/7oz butternut squash, peeled, deseeded and quartered

3½ tbsp olive oil

60g/2oz (3½ tbsp) unsalted butter, plus 2 tbsp for the *mantecatura*

1.2 litres/40fl oz (5 cups) hot onion-free vegetable stock

350g/12oz (scant 1¾ cups) carnaroli, arborio or vialone Nano rice

60g/2oz (½ cup) freshly grated Parmesan cheese

good-quality aged balsamic vinegar, for drizzling

○ ○ ○

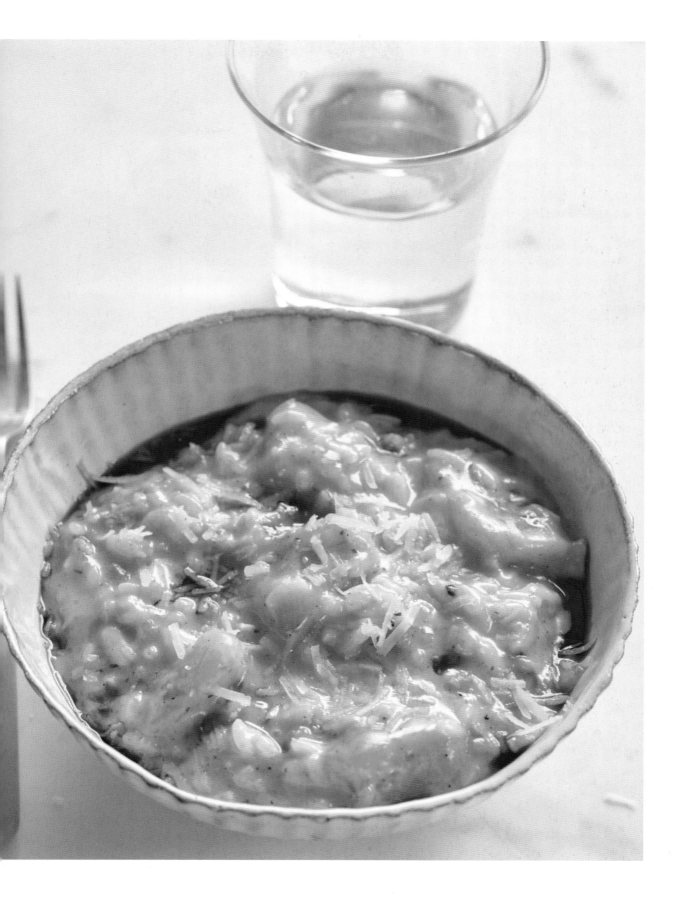

BUTTERNUT SQUASH RISOTTO

1. Cut each quarter of butternut squash into 3mm/⅛in slices — use a sharp knife or a mandolin.

2. Heat the oil and butter in a large heavy-based saucepan over a low heat. Cook the squash for 2–3 minutes, turning a few times, and then add 240ml/8fl oz (1 cup) of the hot vegetable stock (keep it simmering in a pan while you make the risotto). Cook for 15–20 minutes until the squash is tender and starts to fall apart.

3. Add the rice and keep stirring until it absorbs the stock and then add another ladleful. Keep stirring and adding more stock, as and when necessary, in this way until the rice is cooked and just tender (*al dente*) and the risotto has a moist, loose consistency. Be patient and don't try to hurry it — you may be stirring for up to 20 minutes or so.

4. Remove the pan from the heat and beat in the remaining butter and Parmesan (what the Italians call the *mantecatura*). Keep beating with a wooden spoon until the risotto is really glossy and creamy. Check the seasoning and add salt and pepper if necessary — if the stock is well seasoned you probably won't need them.

5. Ladle the risotto into 4 deep plates and drizzle with a little aged balsamic vinegar.

OR YOU CAN TRY THIS…

- Add a small glass of white wine or dry vermouth with the stock.

- Stir in some chopped parsley or chives at the end.

- Sprinkle with more Parmesan and omit the balsamic vinegar.

AUBERGINE &
SPINACH PASANDA

This deliciously rich creamy curry is thickened with ground nuts and coconut milk, which is more FODMAP friendly than dairy cream, and gives the curry a lovely coconut flavour. As this dish is very rich, it is best served with plain boiled rice and a simple vegetable accompaniment.

SERVES 4
PREP: 20 MIN
COOK: 10–20 MIN

60g/2oz blanched almonds

3 tbsp sesame seeds

5cm/2in piece fresh root ginger, peeled and roughly chopped

3 tbsp garlic-infused olive oil

2 tsp ground cumin

2 tsp ground coriander

½ tsp ground turmeric

½ tsp ground cardamom

½ tsp ground cloves

1 tsp ground asafoetida

2 large aubergines (eggplants), cut into 2.5cm/1in cubes

3 tbsp ghee or vegetable oil

400g/14oz can coconut milk

250g/9oz spinach leaves, thick stalks picked off

1 large handful coriander (cilantro), roughly chopped

2 tbsp lemon juice

salt

cooked basmati rice, to serve

1. Put the almonds in a heavy-based frying pan and dry-fry over a gentle heat until just golden brown. Remove from the pan and leave to cool. Toast the sesame seeds in the same way; allow to cool.

2. Tip the nuts into a blender or food processor and process briefly until finely chopped. Add the sesame seeds, ginger and garlic-infused oil and work to a purée.

3. Set a large saucepan or flameproof casserole over a medium heat. Add the nut puree and cook over a moderately high heat for 2 minutes.

4. Add the ground spices and cook, stirring, for 2 minutes. Add the aubergines and ghee or vegetable oil and cook over a high heat, turning constantly until beginning to brown.

5. Add the coconut milk and season with salt to taste. Bring slowly to the boil, then lower the heat and simmer very gently, covered, for about 20 minutes or until the aubergine is tender and the sauce is reduced. Stir occasionally to prevent the sauce catching on the bottom of the pan.

6. Stir the spinach and coriander into the curry and let the spinach wilt down in the hot sauce. Stir in the lemon juice and check the seasoning. Serve with plain rice.

DESSERTS
&
BAKING

CHOCOLATE YOGHURT-COATED STRAWBERRIES

These fabulous yoghurt-coated frozen strawberries can be eaten as a dessert or a snack. You can make them hours or even a few days in advance and leave in the freezer until you're ready to serve them.

SERVES 4 FOR DESSERT
PREP: 15 MIN, PLUS 1–2 HOURS FREEZING
COOK: 5 MIN

400g/14oz strawberries, with stalks intact
225g/8oz (1 cup) 0% fat Greek yoghurt
110g/4oz (scant ¾ cup) dark (bittersweet) chocolate chips

1. Holding each strawberry by the stalk, lift the leaves up and away from the fruit. Dip the pointed fruit end into a shallow bowl of Greek yoghurt. Leave a little area of red showing around the stalk and leaves at the top.

2. Arrange the dipped strawberries, stalk-side down and yoghurt tip-side up, on a wire rack that will fit inside the freezer. Alternatively, space them out on a baking tray (cookie sheet), lined with parchment or waxed paper.

3. Place in the freezer and leave for at 1–2 hours until the yoghurt is frozen hard. If you have any yoghurt left over, you can dip the frozen strawberries again and return them to the freezer for another hour.

4. When you're ready to serve the strawberries, put the chocolate chips in a heatproof basin and suspend it over a pan of barely simmering water. Leave until the chocolate melts.

5. Remove the frozen strawberries from the freezer and divide them between 4 shallow bowls. Drizzle the melted chocolate over the top and serve immediately.

6. Alternatively, place the individual strawberries on a wire rack or lined tray and drizzle with the melted chocolate and then replace in the freezer. Eat as and when required.

OR YOU CAN TRY THIS…

⊙ Add a couple of drops of vanilla extract to the Greek yoghurt.

⊙ Use blueberries instead of strawberries or a mixture of the two.

⊙ Use white or milk (semisweet) chocolate instead of dark (bittersweet).

CHOCOLATE RASPBERRY ROULADE

A very rich and decadent dessert for a special occasion, this classic roulade is gluten-free. If you prefer not to use whipped cream for the filling, you can substitute virtually fat-free fromage frais or thick Greek yoghurt.

SERVES 8
PREP: 25 MIN
COOK: 15 MIN

180g/6oz dark (bitter-sweet) chocolate (minimum 70% cocoa solids)

5 medium free-range eggs, separated

150g/5oz (generous ½ cup) caster (superfine) sugar

300ml/10½fl oz (1¼ cups) double (heavy) lactose-free cream

250g/9oz (2 cups) fresh raspberries

icing (confectioner's) sugar, for dusting

1. Preheat the oven to 180°C, 350°F, gas mark 4. Line a shallow 30 x 23cm/12 x 9in Swiss roll tin (jelly roll pan) with baking parchment.

2. Break the chocolate into pieces and put them in a heatproof bowl suspended over a pan of simmering water. When they melt, remove the bowl from the heat and stir in 3 tablespoons of the hot water in the pan to slacken the melted chocolate.

3. Using an electric whisk, beat the egg yolks with the sugar until really pale, thick and fluffy – be patient, this will take about 5 minutes. Beat into the melted chocolate.

⊙ ⊙ ⊙

···CHOCOLATE RASPBERRY ROULADE

4. In another clean dry bowl, whisk the egg whites until they form stiff peaks. Fold gently into the chocolate mixture with a metal spoon, using a figure-of-eight motion. You want to mix it in thoroughly so there are no visible white clumps of egg white, but taking care not to overdo it so you knock out the air you've beaten in.

5. Pour the mixture into the prepared tin and bake in the preheated oven for about 15 minutes until firm and the top springs back when lightly pressed. Cover with a damp tea towel (dish towel). Leave to cool.

6. Invert the roulade onto a sheet of baking parchment dusted with icing sugar. Peel off the backing paper.

7. Whip the cream until it stands in soft peaks and spread over the roulade, leaving a small border around the edge. Scatter the raspberries over the top and roll up the roulade tightly, using the sugared paper to help you. Place, seam-side down, on a serving plate and dust with icing sugar.

8. Serve the roulade cut into slices. Store in an airtight container in the fridge for up to 2 days.

OR YOU CAN TRY THIS…

- Use blueberries or quartered strawberries instead of raspberries.

- Dust with cocoa instead of icing sugar.

- Serve at Christmas as a Yule log dusted with cinnamon sugar and decorated with a sprig of holly leaves.

ORANGE & CARDAMOM CAKE

This unfussy cake with its crunchy topping is unbelievably easy to make and you don't have to spend time decorating it. The cardamom adds a sweet, subtly spicy flavour and aroma.

SERVES 8
PREP: 15 MIN
COOK: 45–50 MIN

10 cardamom pods

180g/6oz (¾ cup) butter, plus extra for greasing

180g/6oz (heaped ¾ cup) golden caster (superfine) sugar

4 medium free-range eggs

grated zest of 2 unwaxed oranges

110g/4oz (generous 1 cup) gluten-free self-raising (self-rising) flour

60g/2oz (generous ¼ cup) ground almonds

juice of 1 orange

2–3 tbsp milk

FOR THE ORANGE DRIZZLE:

2 tbsp demerara (turbinado or golden granulated) sugar

juice of 1 orange

1. Crush the cardamom pods in a pestle and mortar to extract the seeds. Discard the husks and then crush the seeds. Set aside.

2. Preheat the oven to 180°C, 350°F, gas mark 4. Lightly butter a 900g (2lb) loaf tin (pan) and line with baking parchment.

3. In a food processor or with an electric hand-held whisk, beat together the butter and sugar until light and fluffy. Beat in the eggs, one a time, and then add the orange zest, cardamom seeds, flour and ground almonds. Mix in gently on a lower speed and then slacken the mixture (batter) with the orange juice and milk.

4. Transfer the mixture to the prepared loaf tin and level the top. Bake in the preheated oven for 45–50 minutes until risen and golden brown. Test if the cake is cooked by inserting a thin skewer into the centre – it should come out clean. Remove from the oven and pierce the top of the cake all over with a skewer.

5. Make the orange drizzle: stir the sugar into the orange juice. Drizzle over the top of the cake and leave in the tin until completely cool. Store wrapped in kitchen foil in an airtight container for 4–5 days. Serve cut into slices.

OR YOU CAN TRY THIS…

- Add some crushed cardamom seeds to the orange drizzle for extra spice.

- Make this cake with lemons or limes instead of oranges.

STRAWBERRY CRUMBLE

During the summer when strawberries are seasonal and plentiful, this crumble is an unusual and delicious way of enjoying them.

SERVES 4
PREP: 15 MIN
COOK: 30–40 MIN

500g/1lb 2oz strawberries, hulled

grated zest and juice of ½ orange

3 tbsp caster (superfine) sugar

15g/½oz (1 tbsp) butter, diced

lactose-free cream or Greek yoghurt, to serve

FOR THE CRUMBLE TOPPING:

150g/5oz (1½ cups) gluten-free flour

110g/4oz (½ cup) butter, diced

85g/3oz (scant ½ cup) demerara (turbinado) or golden caster (superfine) sugar

60g/2oz (generous ¼ cup) ground almonds

◎ ◎ ◎

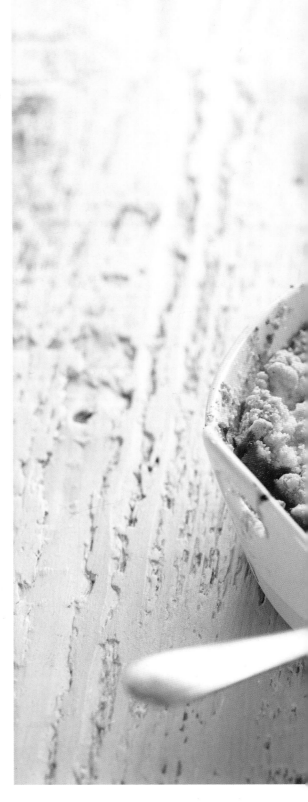

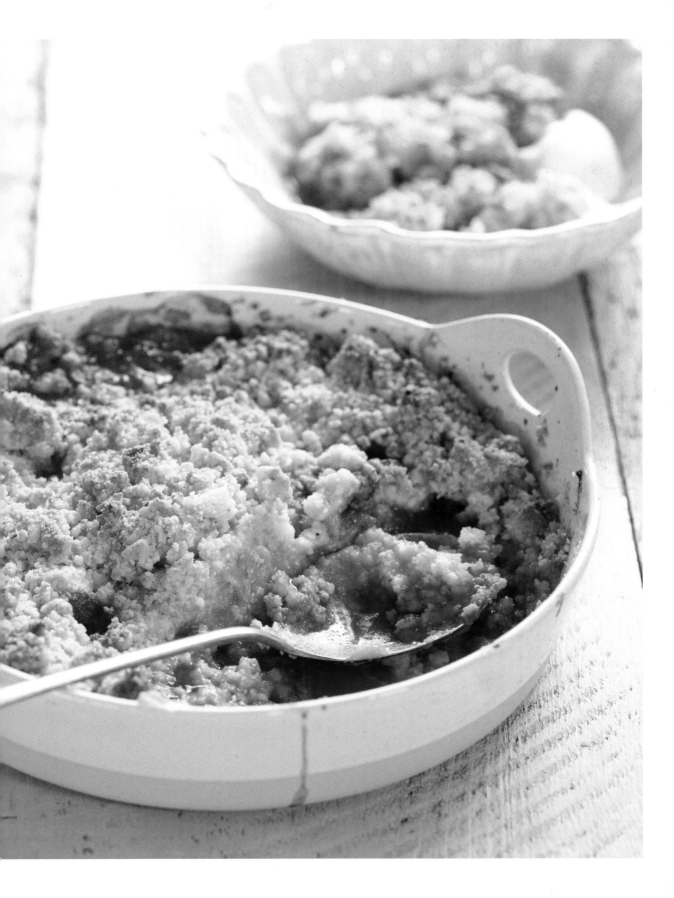

... STRAWBERRY CRUMBLE

1. Preheat the oven to 180°C, 350°F, gas mark 4.

2. Make the crumble topping: put the flour in a large mixing bowl and rub in the butter with your fingertips until the mixture resembles fine breadcrumbs. Stir in the sugar and ground almonds. Add a few drops of water and stir in gently so the mixture clings together a little.

3. Put the strawberries in an ovenproof dish and sprinkle over the orange zest, juice and sugar. Dot the top with butter.

4. Spoon the crumble topping over the strawberries to cover them right up to the edges of the dish. Bake in the preheated oven for 30–40 minutes until the topping is crisp and golden.

5. Serve the hot crumble with cold lactose-free cream or Greek yoghurt.

OR YOU CAN TRY THIS...

- Use raspberries instead of strawberries.

- Use half strawberries and half pink rhubarb cut into chunks. Add extra sugar to counteract the acidity of the rhubarb.

- Substitute lemon zest and juice for the orange.

SQUIDGY CINNAMON MERINGUE CAKE

Really a Pavlova in disguise, this meringue — with its marshmallowy middle — is flavoured with cinnamon and baked in rectangles, then sandwiched together with a light cream and yoghurt filling tossed with chunks of fresh strawberries. It is better assembled an hour or two in advance and allowed to soften slightly. Serve in slices in a pool of cassis-flavoured strawberry sauce.

SERVES 8
PREP: 30 MIN
COOK: 50 MIN

FOR THE MERINGUE:

3 egg whites

180g/6oz (scant 1 cup) caster (superfine) sugar

1 tsp cornflour (cornstarch)

½ tsp ground cinnamon, plus a little to dust

1 tsp lemon juice

FOR THE FILLING:

150ml/5fl oz (⅔ cup) double (heavy) lactose-free cream

150g/5½oz (⅔ cup) Greek yoghurt or lactose-free yoghurt

30g/1oz (2 tbsp) vanilla sugar

350g/12oz strawberries

FOR THE STAWBERRY SAUCE:

450g/1lb strawberries

4 tbsp caster (superfine) sugar

4 tbsp crème de cassis liqueur (optional)

1. Preheat the oven to 150°C, 300°F, gas mark 2. Line two baking (cookie) sheets with non-stick baking parchment. Draw three 11 × 23cm/4½ × 9in rectangles on the paper then turn the paper over so the pencil marks are underneath.

2. Place the egg whites in a large bowl and whisk with an electric beater or large balloon whisk until very stiff. Whisk in the sugar 2 tablespoons at a time, whisking well after each addition until the meringue is stiff and shiny. When all the sugar is incorporated, whisk in the cornflour, cinnamon and lemon juice.

3. Pipe or spoon the meringue mixture on to the rectangles on the prepared baking sheets and spread out to fill them evenly. Place in the oven, reduce the temperature to 140°C, 275°F, gas mark 1 and bake for 50 minutes. Turn off the oven and leave the meringues in the oven until cold.

4. To make the strawberry sauce, either whizz the strawberries in a food processor or blender, then sieve to remove the pips; or simply push them through a fine sieve. Stir in the sugar and liqueur (if using) and chill in the refrigerator until ready to serve.

5. For the filling, whip the cream until holding soft peaks and fold into the Greek yoghurt with the vanilla sugar. Chop the strawberries and fold gently into the cream mixture.

6. To finish, remove the meringues from the baking sheets, carefully peeling off the paper. Sandwich the meringues together with the strawberry filling, then dust the top with a little cinnamon. Serve, cut into slices, on a pool of the strawberry sauce.

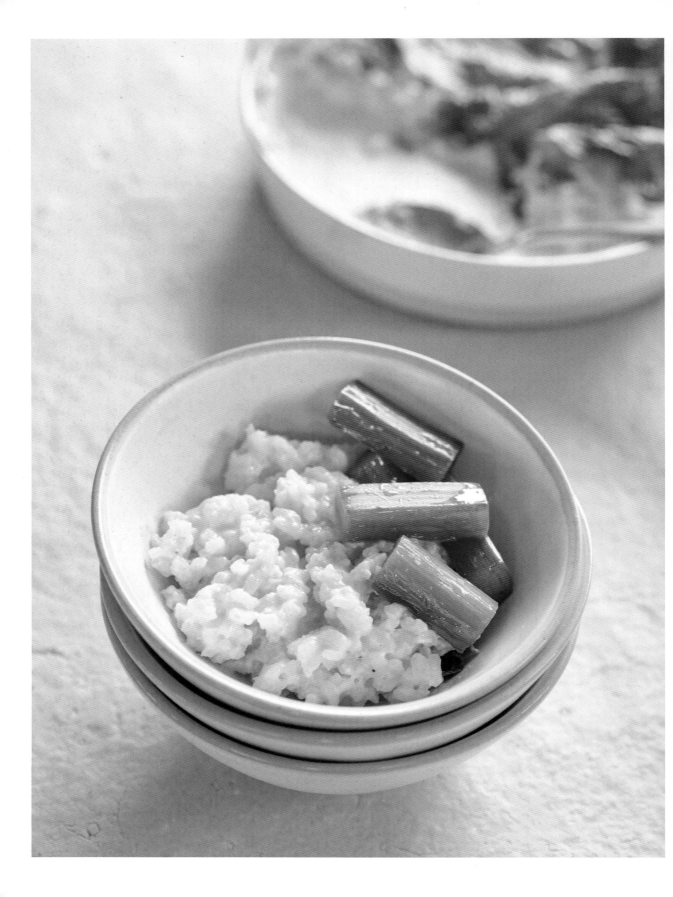

OLD-FASHIONED RICE PUDDING

A bowl of creamy rice pudding, delicately flavoured with warming spices is comfort food at its very best. It's also one of the easiest desserts you'll ever make. It takes just 5 minutes to prepare and then you can pop it into the oven and forget about it for a couple of hours.

SERVES 4
PREP: 5 MIN
COOK: 2 HOURS

85g/3oz (scant ½ cup) short-grain pudding rice (raw weight)

2 tbsp caster (superfine) sugar

600ml/1 pint (2½ cups) whole milk or semi-skimmed milk or nut milk or lactose-free milk

1 cinnamon stick

freshly grated nutmeg

15g/½oz (1 tbsp) butter, cut into tiny pieces, plus extra for greasing

stewed rhubarb, to serve (optional)

OR YOU CAN TRY THIS...

- Instead of a cinnamon stick, add a split vanilla pod (bean) and its seeds.

- Add a bay leaf to the dish before baking.

- For a citrus twist on the traditional pudding, add the grated zest of a lemon or an orange.

- Use risotto rice if you don't have any pudding rice.

- If you have a sweet tooth, serve drizzled with maple syrup.

- Try serving with thick-cut Seville marmalade or jam.

1. Preheat the oven to 150°C, 300°F, gas mark 2. Generously butter a 1 litre/2 pint ovenproof dish.

2. Put the rice and sugar in the dish and pour in the milk. Stir to combine and add the cinnamon stick. Grate the nutmeg over the top and dot with butter.

3. Bake in the preheated oven for 2 hours until the rice is tender, the pudding is thick and creamy and there's a glossy brown skin on top. It's a good idea to check the pudding after about 90 minutes or so, and if it's too thick, to add a little more milk.

4. Remove the cinnamon stick and serve immediately, topped with some stewed rhubarb, if wished.

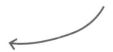

GLUTEN-FREE ZUCCHINI NUT LOAF

This delicious healthy tea-loaf is made with oil instead of butter. Depending on the gluten-free flour you use, you may not need to add the xanthan gum. Check the packet and if it contains xanthan gum, don't add more when you make the loaf.

SERVES 10–12
PREP: 20 MIN
COOK: 1–1¼ HOURS

3 medium free-range eggs

180g/6oz (scant 1 cup) light brown sugar

125ml/4fl oz (½ cup) sunflower oil, plus extra for brushing

300g/10½oz (2 cups) gluten-free flour

½ tsp xanthan gum

1 heaped tsp gluten-free baking powder

½ tsp bicarbonate of soda (baking soda)

1 tsp ground cinnamon

1 tsp ground ginger

½ tsp ground nutmeg

½ tsp salt

3 large courgettes (zucchini), grated

60g/2oz (¼ cup) sultanas (golden raisins)

60g/2oz (scant ½ cup) chopped walnuts

◐ ◐ ◐

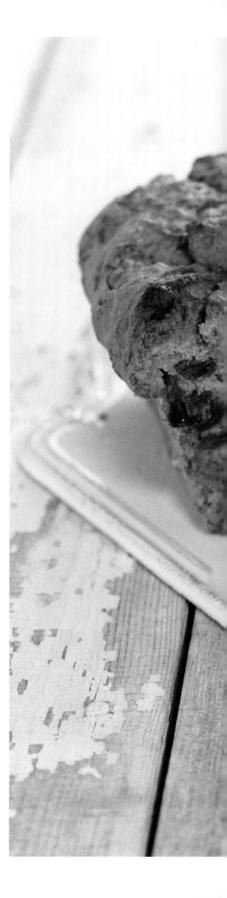

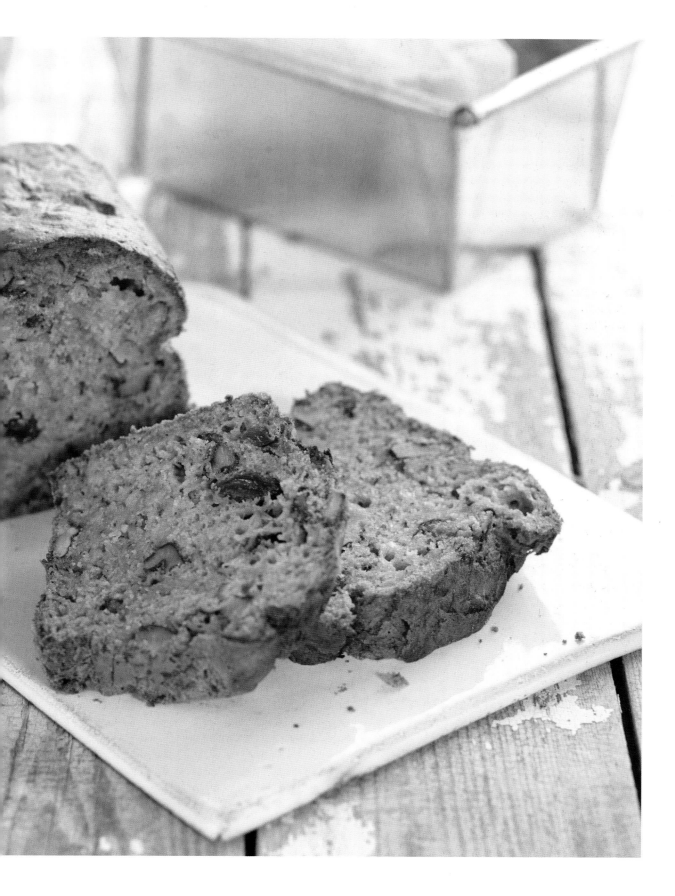

··· GLUTEN-FREE ZUCCHINI NUT LOAF

1. Preheat the oven to 180°C, 350°F, gas mark 4. Lightly oil a 450g/1lb loaf tin (pan) and line with baking parchment.

2. Beat the eggs, sugar and oil in a food mixer or processor until well blended. Mix in the flour, xanthan gum (if using), baking powder, bicarbonate of soda, ground spices and salt on a low speed. Add the grated courgettes and mix in gently with the sultanas and walnuts. If you are using a food processor, stir these in by hand so they don't get blitzed to a pulp.

3. Pour the mixture (batter) into the prepared loaf tin and level the top. Bake in the preheated oven for 1–1¼ hours or until the loaf is well risen and golden brown. Test if it's cooked by inserting a thin skewer into the centre – it should come out clean.

4. Leave the loaf to cool in the tin for 30 minutes before turning it out on to a wire rack. Leave until completely cold.

5. Wrap the loaf in kitchen foil and store in an airtight container in a cool place for up to 3 days – longer in the fridge. Serve cut into slices.

OR YOU CAN TRY THIS...

- Add some diced stem ginger in syrup.
- Flavour with a few drops of vanilla extract.
- Top with soft cheese frosting (see page 240).

LEMON & ROSEMARY POLENTA CAKE

This polenta cake is made with ground hazelnuts instead of the usual almonds to make it FODMAP friendly. You can blitz whole hazelnuts in a spice grinder or food processor if you can't buy ready-ground ones.

SERVES 8
PREP: 15 MIN
COOK: 1 HOUR

150g/5oz (generous ½ cup) butter, plus extra for greasing

150g/5oz (¾ cup) caster (superfine) sugar

3 medium free-range eggs

85g/3oz (1 cup) ground hazelnuts

1 tsp gluten-free baking powder

grated zest and juice of 2 lemons

110g/4oz (scant ¾ cup) ground polenta (cornmeal)

crème fraîche or Greek yoghurt or lactose-free yoghurt, to serve

FOR THE LEMON ROSEMARY SYRUP:
60g/2oz (¼ cup) caster (superfine) sugar

1 tsp finely chopped fresh rosemary leaves

juice of 2 lemons

1. Preheat the oven to 170°C, 325°F, gas mark 3. Lightly butter a 20cm/8in loose-bottomed (springform) cake tin (pan) and line with baking parchment.

2. Beat the butter and sugar together until pale and fluffy. Add the eggs, one at a time, beating well after each addition. Mix in the ground hazelnuts, baking powder and lemon zest. Stir in the lemon juice and polenta.

3. Transfer the mixture to the prepared cake tin and level the top. Bake in the preheated oven for 45–50 minutes until risen and golden brown. Insert a thin skewer to check whether the cake is cooked – it should come out clean. Leave in the tin while you make the syrup.

4. Make the lemon rosemary syrup: put the sugar, rosemary and lemon juice in a small pan and stir over a medium heat until the sugar dissolves. Bring to the boil, then let it bubble away for 4–5 minutes until syrupy and golden.

5. Pierce the cake all over with a thin skewer and slowly pour the lemon rosemary syrup over the top. Leave the cake to cool and soak up the syrup.

6. Serve cut into slices with a spoonful of crème fraîche or yoghurt.

OR YOU CAN TRY THIS...

- Use orange juice and zest instead of lemons.
- Add a dash of vanilla extract to the cake mixture.
- Add some rose water or orange flower water to the syrup.

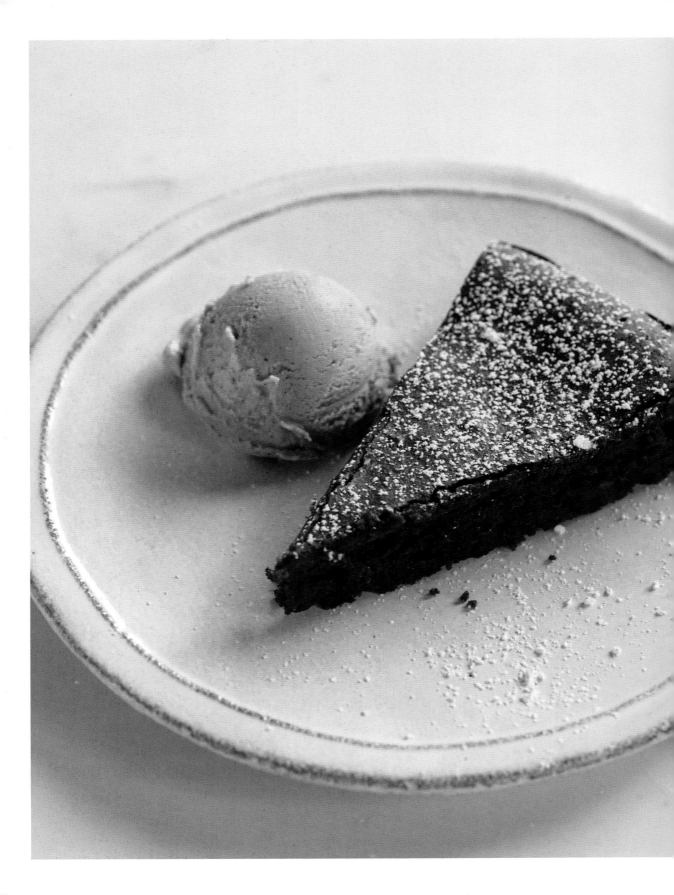

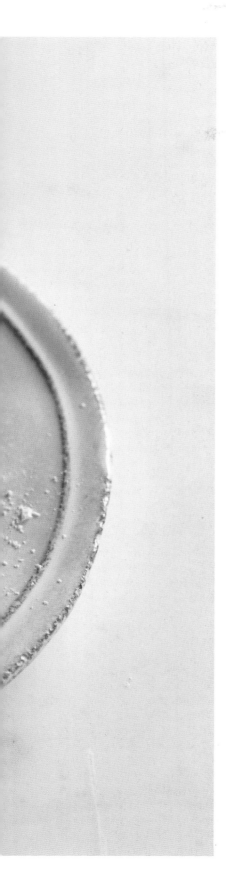

STICKY CHOCOLATE GINGER CAKE

This sticky chocolate cake has a slightly crisp exterior and the soft consistency of a brownie in the centre. You can eat it as a treat or serve it for dessert.

SERVES 8–10
PREP: 20 MIN
COOK: 25 MIN

200g/7oz dark (bitter-sweet) chocolate (minimum 70% cocoa solids)

110g/4oz (½ cup) unsalted butter, diced, plus extra for greasing

4 medium free-range eggs, separated

120g/4½oz (generous ½ cup) caster (superfine) sugar

5 pieces stem ginger in syrup, finely chopped

2 tbsp ginger syrup from the jar

1 tbsp cornflour (cornstarch)

icing (confectioner's sugar) for dusting

1. Preheat the oven to 180°C, 350°F, gas mark 4. Lightly butter a 23cm/9in loose-bottomed (springform) cake tin (pan) and line with parchment paper.

2. Break the chocolate into pieces and put them with the butter in a heatproof bowl suspended over a pan of simmering water. When they melt, remove the bowl from the heat and stir well.

3. Beat the egg yolks with the sugar until really pale and fluffy – be patient, this will take about 5 minutes.

○ ○ ○

...STICKY CHOCOLATE GINGER CAKE

4. In another clean dry bowl, whisk the egg whites until, they form stiff peaks.

5. Fold the melted chocolate and butter into the egg yolk mixture and then stir in the chopped stem ginger, syrup and cornflour. With a metal spoon, fold in the beaten egg white in a figure-of-eight motion. Do this very lightly so as to keep as much air as possible in the cake mixture (batter).

6. Spoon into the prepared tin and bake in the preheated oven for about 25 minutes until the cake is well risen. Test whether it's cooked by inserting a thin skewer – it should come out quite clean but still moist. If the cake is still really sticky, pop it back in the oven for another 5 minutes.

7. Leave the cake to cool a little in the tin and don't worry if it goes down in the middle and cracks a little on top – it's not a sponge cake. Serve slightly warm, dusted with icing sugar and cut into thin slices. Lactose-free ice cream and fresh berries make a great accompaniment if you are serving this as a dessert.

OR YOU CAN TRY THIS...

- Omit the ginger and add the grated zest of 1 orange or a few drops of vanilla extract.

- Use soft brown sugar instead of white.

GRIDDLED FRUIT KEBABS WITH CHOCOLATE DIPPING SAUCE

Everybody will love these juicy kebabs with chocolate sauce, especially children. You can cook them over hot coals on a barbecue in summer.

SERVES 4
PREP: 15 MIN, PLUS SOAKING
COOK: 10 MIN

2 large bananas, thickly sliced

juice of ½ lemon

2 ripe papayas (pawpaw), peeled, deseeded and cubed

4 thick slices pineapple, cubed

1 ripe mango, peeled, stoned (pitted) and cubed

225g/8oz whole strawberries, hulled

¼ tsp ground cinnamon

icing (confectioner's) sugar, for dusting

FOR THE CHOCOLATE DIPPING SAUCE:
150g/5oz dark (bittersweet) chocolate

1 tbsp golden (corn) syrup

120ml/4fl oz (½ cup) lactose-free double (heavy) cream

1. Preheat the grill (broiler). Soak 8 thin wooden or bamboo skewers in warm water for 15–30 minutes to prevent them burning under the hot grill.

2. Brush the sliced banana with lemon juice to prevent it discolouring. Thread the prepared fruit alternately onto the skewers and dust with the ground cinnamon and icing sugar.

3. Place the fruit skewers on a foil-lined grill (broiler) pan and cook under the preheated hot grill for about 5 minutes, turning occasionally, until hot and slightly caramelized but not charred.

4. Meanwhile, make the chocolate dipping sauce: put the chocolate, golden syrup and cream in a small heavy-based pan over a low heat. Warm gently until the chocolate melts, stirring to combine. Remove from the heat and pour into 4 individual little pots or ramekins.

5. Serve the griddled kebabs immediately with the warm chocolate dipping sauce.

OR YOU CAN TRY THIS...
- Add a few drops of vanilla extract to the chocolate dipping sauce.

- Serve the kebabs with lactose-free ice cream or some refreshing sorbet.

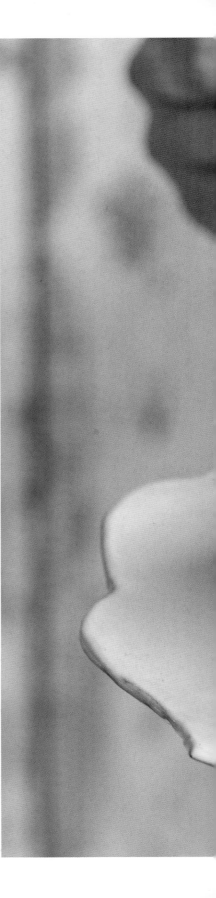

SPICY CARROT & ORANGE CAKE

This cake must be kept fresh in the fridge because of the soft cheese and Quark in the frosting. However, if you prefer it virgin and unadorned, just sprinkle with icing (confectioner's) sugar and it will stay moist stored in an airtight container in a cool place for 5 days.

SERVES 10–12
PREP: 20 MIN
COOK: 40–45 MIN

180g/6oz (¾ cup) caster (superfine) sugar

180ml/6fl oz (¾ cup) sunflower oil

3 medium free-range eggs, beaten

225g/8oz (2 cups) grated carrot

finely grated zest and juice of 1 orange

180g/6oz (generous 1½ cups) gluten-free flour

1 tsp gluten-free baking powder

1 tsp ground cinnamon

½ tsp grated nutmeg

½ tsp ground ginger

60g/2oz (generous ¼ cup) sultanas (golden raisins)

FOR THE FROSTING:
110g/4oz (scant ½ cup) Quark (or thick 0% fat Greek yoghurt or lactose-free thick plain yoghurt)

110g/4oz (½ cup) lactose-free cream cheese

2–3 tbsp icing (confectioner's) sugar

grated zest of 1 orange and a squeeze of orange juice

◦ ◦ ◦

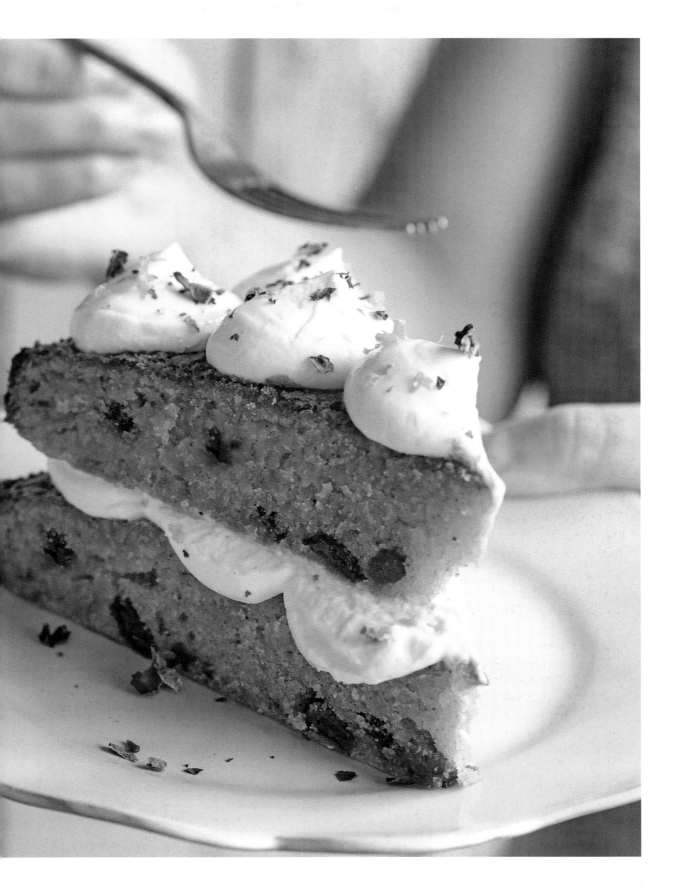

˚˚˚ SPICY CARROT & ORANGE CAKE

1. Preheat the oven to 180°C, 350°F, gas mark 4. Lightly oil a 23cm/9in loose-bottomed (springform) cake tin (pan) and line with baking parchment.

2. In a mixing bowl or food mixer, beat the sugar, oil and eggs until well combined. Mix in the grated carrot and orange zest.

3. Sift in the flour, baking powder and spices and mix well. Stir in the orange juice and sultanas. Spoon the mixture into the prepared cake tin and level the top.

4. Bake in the preheated oven for 40–45 minutes until well risen and a skewer insert into the centre comes out clean. Cool in the tin and then turn out onto a wire rack.

5. Make the frosting: mix together all the ingredients until smooth and creamy. Spread over the top of the cool cake. Store in an airtight container in the fridge. Serve the cake cut into slices.

OR YOU CAN TRY THIS...

- Add a few drops of vanilla extract to the cake mixture.

- Stir in a handful of chopped walnuts or pecans with the sultanas just before baking.

- Make the cake in a 900g/2lb loaf tin (pan) instead of a round cake tin.

BROWN SUGAR MERINGUES
WITH MANGO
& A RASPBERRY SAUCE

Generous clouds of meringue are filled with whipped cream and golden mango chunks and served on a sharp ruby red sauce. Demerara sugar adds a slight caramel flavour to the meringues and colours them a pretty, pale beige.

SERVES 6
PREP: 35 MIN, PLUS COOLING
COOK: 3–4 HOURS

FOR THE MERINGUE:
4 egg whites
110g/4oz (generous ½ cup)
    granulated sugar
110g/4oz (generous ½ cup)
    demerara (turbinado) sugar

FOR THE RASPBERRY SAUCE:
450g/1lb fresh or frozen
    raspberries, thawed
2 tbsp lemon juice
icing (confectioner's) sugar,
    to taste
2 tbsp kirsch

TO ASSEMBLE:
2 ripe mangoes
150ml/5fl oz (⅔ cup) double
    (heavy) lactose-free cream
150ml/5fl oz thick Greek yoghurt
    or lactose-free yoghurt
1 tbsp icing (confectioner's) sugar

1. Preheat the oven to 110°C, 225 °F, gas mark ½. Put the egg whites in a large bowl and whisk until very stiff but not dry. Gradually whisk in the combined sugars, spoonful by spoonful, allowing the mixture to become very stiff between each addition.

2. Line a baking (cookie) sheet with non-stick baking parchment. Spoon or pipe about 12 meringues onto the parchment. Bake in the oven for 3–4 hours until thoroughly dried out.

3. Remove the meringues from the oven and leave to cool on the parchment. Carefully lift off when cool and store in an airtight container until required.

4. To make the raspberry sauce, place the raspberries in a blender or food processor with the lemon juice and icing sugar to taste. Work to a purée, then pass through a sieve to remove any seeds. Stir in the kirsch, cover and chill in the refrigerator.

5. Cut the flesh from the mangoes, then remove the skin and cut into slices.

6. To serve, whip the cream until it just holds soft peaks, then fold in the yoghurt and icing sugar. Spoon the cream onto six of the meringues. Arrange the sliced mango on top and sandwich together with the remaining meringues. Place on individual serving plates and pour over the raspberry sauce. Serve immediately.

DARK CHOCOLATE & RASPBERRY BREAD & BUTTER PUDDING

This recipe uses a lovely toasted almond milk for extra flavour. Combined with cinnamon, dark chocolate and raspberries, it's a moreish combination.

SERVES 4–6
PREP: 20 MIN, PLUS SOAKING
COOK: 30 MIN

200g/7oz sliced gluten-free bread

about 40g/1½oz (3 tbsp) butter, for spreading

60g/2oz dark chocolate chunks

100g/3½oz raspberries

3 eggs

300ml/10½fl oz (1¼ cups) roasted almond milk

100ml/3½fl oz (scant 1 cup) double (heavy) lactose-free cream

60g/2oz (¼ cup) caster (superfine) sugar, plus extra to sprinkle

1 tsp ground cinnamon

1. Butter the bread slices on both sides and slice them twice diagonally into small triangles. Lay one layer flat into a baking dish and sprinkle over most of the chocolate and raspberries. Arrange the remaining triangles, over the top in an attractive pattern, and scatter over the remaining chocolate and raspberries.

2. In a bowl, beat the eggs lightly, then add the almond milk, cream, sugar and cinnamon and mix well to combine.

3. Pour the liquid over the bread in the dish and gently push the bread down to make sure all the bread has been dampened by the milk. Go gently here as gluten-free bread is not quite as sturdy as wheat bread, and so it may start to break up. Leave to sit so that the bread can absorb the milk for 30 minutes or so. Meanwhile, preheat the oven to 190°C, 375°F, gas mark 5.

4. Sprinkle sugar over the top of the pudding and bake for 30–35 minutes, until golden brown and crisp on top and set underneath, then serve straightaway while the chocolate is still melted.

RASPBERRY & COCOA SORBETS

This duo of sorbets tastes as exciting as it looks. Dark chocolate makes a surprisingly good sorbet – cocoa is used here to give a wonderfully intense flavour. The refreshing raspberry sorbet provides a fantastic colour and flavour contrast.

SERVES 6
PREP: 40 MIN, PLUS FREEZING
COOK: 5 MIN

FOR THE CHOCOLATE SORBET:
40g/1½oz (4 tbsp) cocoa powder

100g/3½oz (½ cup) granulated sugar

1 tsp vanilla extract

1 egg white

FOR THE RASPBERRY SORBET:
180g/6oz (scant 1 cup) caster (superfine) sugar

450g/1lb raspberries

juice of 2 lemons

1 egg white

TO SERVE:
110g/4oz raspberries

lemon balm or mint leaves,
    to decorate

icing (confectioners') sugar,
    for dusting

⊙ ⊙ ⊙

··· RASPBERRY & COCOA SORBETS

1. To make the chocolate sorbet, place the cocoa powder, sugar and 480ml/16fl oz (2 cups) water in a heavy-based saucepan. Dissolve over a low heat, stirring occasionally, then bring to the boil and boil for 2 minutes, without stirring. Remove from the heat, stir in the vanilla extract and leave to cool.

2. Pour the cocoa mixture into a freezer-proof container and freeze for 2–3 hours until slushy. Whisk the egg white until holding soft peaks. Whizz the sorbet in a food processor, or tip into a bowl and beat well, then fold in the egg white. Return to the freezer container, cover and freeze for 3–4 hours until firm.

3. To make the raspberry sorbet, place the sugar in a saucepan with 150ml/5fl oz (⅔ cup) water and dissolve over a low heat, stirring occasionally, then bring to the boil and boil for 2 minutes, without stirring.

4. Whizz the raspberries in a food processor or blender, add the syrup and process again, then sieve to remove the pips. Add the lemon juice and leave to cool. Pour into a freezerproof container, then freeze for 2–3 hours until slushy. Whisk the egg white until holding soft peaks. Briefly process or beat the sorbet, then fold in the egg white. Return to container, cover and freeze until firm.

5. To serve, transfer the sorbets to the refrigerator for 20 minutes to soften, then arrange balls of alternate flavours on individual serving plates. Scatter with raspberries and lemon balm or mint leaves. Dust with icing sugar and serve at once.

RHUBARB & GINGER ICE CREAM

Rhubarb and ginger is a truly tried-and-tested favourite combination. The ice cream can be pale pink or green depending on the type of rhubarb – adding a drop of natural food colouring enhances the colour. Dainty ginger biscuits are the perfect complement, and making them with rice flour makes them beautifully crisp.

SERVES 4
PREP: 45 MIN, PLUS FREEZING
COOK: 40 MIN

350g/12oz trimmed rhubarb stalks

60g/2oz (¼ cup) golden caster sugar, or to taste

2 tbsp ginger syrup from the jar, plus more if needed

210ml/7fl oz (scant 1 cup) double (heavy) lactose-free cream

2 egg yolks

100ml/3½fl oz (scant ½ cup) Greek yoghurt or lactose-free yoghurt

85g/3oz stem ginger in syrup, drained and finely sliced

FOR THE GINGER BISCUITS

60 g/2oz (3½ tbsp) butter

30g/1oz (⅛ cup) caster sugar, plus extra for dusting

60g/2oz (⅓ cup) white rice flour

30g/1oz (3 tbsp) cornflour (cornstarch)

1 tsp ground ginger

1. Cut the rhubarb into chunks and place in a saucepan with the sugar and ginger syrup. Bring to the boil, lower the heat and simmer for 15–20 minutes until very tender. Allow to cool slightly, then purée in a blender or food processor until smooth.

2. Pour the cream into a saucepan and bring to the boil. Whisk the egg yolks together in a bowl, then whisk in the scalded cream. Return to the pan and add the rhubarb purée. Stir the rhubarb custard over a very gentle heat for about 10 minutes until thickening. Remove from the heat, cover the surface with greaseproof paper to prevent a skin forming and allow to cool, then chill.

3. Stir the yoghurt and stem ginger into the chilled rhubarb custard, then taste and add more ginger syrup if necessary. Freeze in an ice cream machine, according to the manufacturer's directions. Alternatively, turn into a freezerproof container, cover and freeze until firm, whisking occasionally (see note).

⊙ ⊙ ⊙

RHUBARB
& GINGER ICE CREAM

4. To make the ginger biscuits, cream the butter and sugar together in a bowl. Sift the flours and ginger together over the mixture, then beat in thoroughly. When the mixture forms a ball, knead lightly, then roll out on a floured surface to a 3mm (⅛ in) thickness. Using a 6cm/2½in round cookie cutter, cut out 8 rounds and place on a baking sheet that has been lined with baking paper. Chill for 15 minutes.

5. Preheat the oven to 190°C, 375°F, gas mark 5, then bake the biscuits for 10–15 minutes, or until light golden. Sprinkle with caster sugar whilst still warm. Leave to cool.

6. Scoop the ice cream into serving dishes and serve with 2 ginger biscuits per person.

NOTE: If you are not using an ice cream maker, it is important to whisk the mixture periodically during freezing to break down the ice crystals and ensure a smooth-textured result.

COCONUT ICE CREAM

Coconuts are plentiful all over India and are used extensively in sweet and savoury dishes. Although this recipe isn't a true ice cream, it makes a simple refreshing dessert to follow a spicy main course. The edible rose petal decoration is optional, but provides a stunning contrast to the gleaming white ice cream.

SERVES 8
PREP: 15 MIN, PLUS FREEZING
COOK: 10 MIN

275g/10oz (heaped 1¼ cup) granulated sugar

4 x 400ml/14oz cans coconut milk

TO DECORATE (OPTIONAL):
a few dark red rose petals

a few shredded dried red rose petals

freshly grated nutmeg

ground cinnamon

1. Set the freezer to fast-freeze. Put the sugar with 600ml/1 pint (2½ cups) water in a medium heavy-based saucepan and dissolve over a medium heat, stirring occasionally. As soon as it is dissolved, stop stirring, increase the heat and boil rapidly for 10 minutes to make a sugar syrup. Leave to cool completely.

2. Blend the cooled syrup with the coconut milk. Pour into a shallow freezerproof container, cover and freeze for about 3 hours or until partially frozen.

3. Spoon the mixture into a blender or food processor and quickly blend on high speed to break down the ice crystals without letting the ice cream melt. Immediately return to the container, recover and freeze again just until mushy. This will probably take another 2 hours.

4. Tip the ice cream into the blender or processor and process again as before. Return to the container, cover tightly and freeze for about 3 hours until firm. The ice cream is now ready to eat.

5. Remove the ice cream from the freezer and leave for 10–20 minutes at cool room temperature to soften before serving.

6. Scoop the ice cream into serving dishes. Scatter with the rose petals, nutmeg and cinnamon if using.

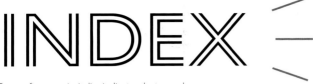

INDEX

Page references in *italics* indicate photographs.

RESOURCES
& USEFUL INFORMATION

WEBSITES

IBS Diets
Dieting guide with information and FODMAP
food lists.
www.ibsdiets.org

The IBS Network
The UK's national charity for IBS, offering
information, advice and support to people
living with Irritable Bowel Syndrome.
www.theibsnetwork.org

The Monash University Low FODMAP Diet
Information on high and low FODMAP foods,
latest research, food lists, etc.
www.med.monash.edu.au

APPS

King's College London FODMAP app
Includes latest news, research and information
on the low FODMAP diet.
www.kcl.ac.uk

Low FODMAP smartphone app
The Monash University Low FODMAP Diet
App helps you to follow the diet and manage
your symptoms
www.med.monash.edu.au

BIBLIOGRAPHY

The Complete Low FODMAP Diet
Dr Sue Shepherd and Dr Peter Gibson
(Vermilion 2014)

The Low FODMAP Diet Cookbook
Dr Sue Shepherd (Vermilion 2015)